MORAL CONFLICTS
OF ORGAN RETRIEVAL

A Case for Constructive Pluralism

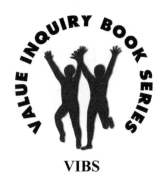

VIBS

Volume 172

Robert Ginsberg
Founding Editor

Peter A. Redpath
Executive Editor

Associate Editors

a volume in
Values in Bioethics
ViB
Matti Häyry and Tuija Takala, Editors

MORAL CONFLICTS
OF ORGAN RETRIEVAL
A Case for Constructive Pluralism

Charles C. Hinkley II

Amsterdam - New York, NY 2005

Cover Design: Studio Pollmann

The paper on which this book is printed meets the requirements of "ISO 9706:1994, Information and documentation - Paper for documents - Requirements for permanence".

ISBN: 90-420-1737-6
©Editions Rodopi B.V., Amsterdam - New York, NY 2005
Printed in the Netherlands

CONTENTS

FOREWORD

We have the capability to prolong people's lives by replacing defective organs with those of other people and non-human animals. We approach a time when we can create organs needed for transplants from the stem cells of embryos. We feel obligated to prolong and improve people's lives with organ transplants while at the same showing due respect to the donors, providers, and sellers, living or dead. How should we proceed? What are the best alternatives? What happens when the worlds of medicine and ethics collide?

Charles Hinkley acquaints us fully with the rich literature on the subject, the issues and value conflicts that arise, and the range of answers commentators have offered. We learn about the routine retrieval of some organs from the newly dead and how professionals assume consent in some situations. We become acquainted with how competing conceptions of death affect the retrieval and transplantation of organs. We see how controversial issues surround matters like these. Can we wrong the dead? Do we wrong the dead when we presume consent? Who are the dead?

Throughout the work, Hinkley demonstrates how conflicting values and our sacrificing one to the other leads to regret and guilt. He joins those commentators who urge us to avoid these situations when we can but goes much further as he takes a fresh look at our moral lives. He argues for their being creative endeavors that offer alternatively viable resolutions to these conflicts that provide occasions for moral growth. In this way, *The Moral Conflicts of Organ Retrieval* ingeniously advances our thinking about the ethics of organ transplantation as it does so for the field of ethics itself.

Vincent Luizzi
Texas State University–San Marcos
San Marcos, Texas

ACKNOWLEDGMENTS

Biggest thanks go to my mother, Edith Holland, and my wife Suzannah for their support. Special thanks to Vincent Luizzi for his friendship, and for suggesting that I address the central themes of constructive pluralism earlier in the book.

Matti Häyry and Tuija Takala deserve credit for many helpful suggestions. The following individuals were helpful with editing and proofreading: Douglas Anderson, Peter Redpath, Eric van Broekhuizen, Peter Herissone-Kelly, Jeannie Bruton, Kayhan Parsi, Jerry Worley, and Ronnie DeVries. Beverly Pairett, and Elizabeth Boepple deserve much credit for bringing this manuscript to the point of being camera ready. Elizabeth's familiarity with the Value Inquiry Book Series specifications proved invaluable.

Early discussions with several individuals at the University of Texas Medical Branch at Galveston, most notably Bill Winslade and John Douard, proved helpful. Thanks to Pearl Cox for sharing her experience as a kidney transplant recipient. Thanks to my sisters Shauna Jacobson, Andrea Holland, Yoland Hinkley, and Sam Bender for helpful discussions. Thanks also to my philosophy students at Texas State University–San Marcos for their helpful remarks on an earlier draft of the introduction. Melody Pace provided helpful research assistance.

INTRODUCTION

The medical-scientific-bioethical community and the lay public bemoan the scarcity of transplantable organs. Although more than 24,000 people in the United States received an organ transplant in 2003, more than 6,000 others died while waiting for one.[1] Increasing the donor pool through innocuous measures such as education and sympathetic appeals is insufficient. Consequently, scholars debate remedial but controversial proposals: (1) salvage organs as needed; (2) presume individuals wish to donate unless they explicitly indicate otherwise; (3) alter the criteria for determining death; (4) transplant animal organs into humans; (4) offer financial incentives to potential donors; (5) develop promising research on stem cells including cells taken from embryos and fetuses that may lead to the repair or creation of organs. The quest for organs, then, creates apparent value conflicts between extending life for patients with failing organs and treating decedents, the dying, animals, persons and their bodies, embryos, and fetuses with proper moral regard. In this book, I identify the value conflicts generated by our practices and proposals to retrieve more organs, explore the moral ramifications of these conflicts, and develop an interpretation and response that I call constructive pluralism.

This book consists of three major parts. Part One has three chapters that provide a philosophical framework in which to interpret and evaluate moral conflicts and conflicts with organ retrieval. Chapter one addresses the nature and implications of moral conflict. Chapter two covers different approaches to medical ethics including the dominant model of medical ethics in the United States. I focus on American medical ethics only because that is the tradition with which I am most familiar. Chapter three pertains to issues related to comparing and weighing the value of our options. Part Two contains one chapter summarizing the quality of life of transplant patients and five chapters that address the moral conflicts of organ retrieval strategies involving the moral status of decedents, redefining death, selling organs, animal transplants, and stem cell research. Part Three consists of two chapters that address how we ought to respond to organ retrieval conflicts. Chapter ten addresses the extent to which we ought to avoid conflicts. The final chapter sets forth in more detail the meaning of constructive pluralism for assessing organ retrieval strategies. Readers should understand that while I attempt to address issues with organ transplantation, my primary purpose is to illuminate ethics through the study of organ transplantation.

In chapter one, I examine a rich philosophical literature about conflicting values that produce a negative aftermath. Even if we make justifiable or excellent choices in times of conflict, acting based on one value often means failing to realize, or, perhaps, violating the dictates of other values. Conflicts can make bad consequences inevitable, or make any action taken appear to constitute wrongdoing; conflicts can leave us with moral losses no matter how well we respond to them. In turn, moral losses provide the basis for moral residue including regret, guilt, or requirements to apologize, make amends, offer explanations, or avoid some kinds of future conflicts.[2] Hereafter, I sometimes use "residue" for moral residue.

The implications of residue remain controversial. Does residue imply the existence of dilemmas—situations wherein we face two or more requirements that cannot both be satisfied? If so, since failing to satisfy our requirements suggests wrongdoing and blameworthiness, dilemmas necessitate that we morally fail. No matter our good intentions and efforts, we can be condemned to wrongdoing that warrants blame or taints us. Believing that some conflicts leave residue without also implying dilemmas leaves us with an explanatory problem. How can residual requirements exist if a conflict did not involve more than one requirement? Whether dilemmas exist in this sense, the debates over dilemmas pave the way for understanding many conflicts in the quest for organs as residue-producing conflicts. To explain organ retrieval conflicts, I address how United States commentators often approach ethical conflicts in medicine.

In chapter two, I discuss five approaches to medical ethics. The first approach is Tom Beauchamp and James Childress's four-principle model.[3] Second, Edmund Pellegrino and David Thomasma offer a model based on virtue ethics.[4] Feminist ethics is the third approach. Fourth, Albert R. Jonsen, Mark Siegler, and William J. Winslade present a case-based approach.[5] The fifth model is Hugo Tristram Engelhardt's postmodern libertarianism.[6] The model of Beauchamp and Childress has had the greatest influence on American medical ethics and will receive greater attention.

Beauchamp and Childress set forth four principles based on the value of individual autonomy, beneficence, nonmaleficence, and justice that guide us in determining what should be done regarding different issues in medical ethics. They harbor no illusions that their model is set in stone or capable of providing the basis to answer all questions in medical ethics. They explicitly claim that our beliefs about ethics are limited, sometimes incoherent, and subject to revision.[7] Interestingly, the American medical ethics community, especially the work of healthcare providers, has religiously adopted their four principles, but has not seriously considered their views on the limitations of moral concepts and the need to make revisions among our beliefs.

In contrast to Beauchamp and Childress, Pellegrino and Thomasma offer a medical ethics model based on virtue ethics. They attempt to supplement Beauchamp and Childress's model for two primary reasons. First, virtuous persons will be more inclined to follow principles. Second, Pellegrino and Thomasma believe that the cultivation of virtuous character increases our chances of making the right decision in difficult circumstances.

Feminist bioethicists such as Rosemarie Tong and Susan Sherwin emphasize that making ethical decisions must include the political and historical context of the moral problem in question.[8] We should closely examine the relationships of those involved with moral decision-making in terms of power relations between decision-makers and those affected by the decisions. The goal of feminist ethics is to overcome oppressive practices, especially those contributing to the subordination of women, and to foster freely chosen relationships that people find enriching. Unfortunately, feminist bioethicists have not devoted much attention to organ transplantation.

Jonsen, Siegler, and Winslade demonstrate the efficacy of utilizing the Beauchamp and Childress approach to medical ethics, even though they aim to contrast their case-based approach with the principle model of Beauchamp and Childress. By paying close attention to the contextual details of clinical cases, Jonsen, Siegler, and Winslade believe we can find the best answer to ethical problems that arise in the clinic. The skepticism mentioned by Beauchamp and Childress has no obvious role in Jonsen, Siegler, and Winslade's exposition of clinical ethics. Their confidence in finding moral answers may stem from their focus on clinical cases instead of policy questions, specially selected clinical cases that are resolvable, or on deeper and perhaps unconscious assumptions about moral knowledge. Part of the difficulty with understanding their confidence in finding moral answers results from their failure to clarify what it means to resolve a case. It could mean that relevant parties discover moral answers resulting in agreement, or that parties reach agreement and consider that an answer. Jonsen, Siegler, and Winslade exemplify the optimism that concepts of medical ethics, borrowed largely from Beauchamp and Childress, are sufficient for us to find answers, or provide us with the wherewithal to reach agreements.

Three reasons explain this confidence in finding moral answers to questions related to medical ethics. First, Beauchamp and Childress have provided us with an understandable and user-friendly model of moral deliberation that gives us reason to be confident when considering many significant medical decisions. Second, although Beauchamp and Childress mention problems with inconsistencies in our moral beliefs and the need to make revisions, they do not emphasize that the application of their model will frequently lead to indeterminate or unsatisfactory results. Third, most medical ethicists and laypersons have a strong impulse to find the best answer to moral questions. Not surprisingly, medical ethicists believe that they often find the single best answer to a moral question.

The failure to seriously consider Beauchamp and Childress's remarks on our moral limitations has resulted in a medical ethics often too optimistic that our moral concepts are sufficient for finding answers to all or most moral questions. Whether medical ethicists explicitly accept or reject Beauchamp and Childress's model, widely shared presumptions dictate the shape of medical ethics in the United States. We arrive at answers by accumulating relevant facts, identifying the values involved, factoring in the probability that we can accomplish our goals, balancing conflicting values by weighing our options, and then rendering a judgment. Answers will not always be easily determined or uncontroversial, but medical ethicists with different areas of expertise tend to be confident that determinate answers can be discovered, virtually always a single answer for a policy or case study. I refer to Beauchamp and Childress's four principles conjoined with the assumption that medical ethics questions have single determinate answers as conventional medical ethics.

Conventional medical ethics is understandable and includes necessary features of good decision-making, but it has obvious limitations when applied to organ retrieval. First, the intrinsic value of many potential sources of organs is contentious, for example, dead people, individuals who might be dead, the nearly dead, animals, embryos, and fetuses. This creates a serious problem for identifying the values involved; a problem that many scholars have recognized and addressed. Second, we must make decisions in the light of scientific hopes and facts; witness stem cell research and xenotransplantation. Third, conventional medical ethics fails to characterize the dynamic nature of the moral life that leading moral lives requires persistent effort to create conditions whereby we can fulfill our duties and bring about good consequences. Fourth, we must sometimes decide among incommensurable alternatives, alternatives that resist adequate comparisons for the sake of balancing and ranking the value of our options. With few exceptions, making decisions in the light of incommensurable values is an overlooked issue in medical ethics.

Engelhardt is one of the few American medical ethicists who have addressed the problem of rationally weighing and ranking the value of our options. His skepticism runs deep. He believes that we cannot find ultimate answers to moral questions. According to him, we can agree to negotiate peaceably and consent to solutions to our moral problems. We cannot discover the answers, because of the limitations of our moral knowledge, a view supported, he thinks, by unyielding debate on some moral issues. The inability to find foundations for our moral beliefs lies at the heart of Engelhardt's moral skepticism and explains his turn to moral consensus as constituting what it means to reach a moral resolution in the secular sphere. He regards individual autonomy as necessary and sufficient for consensus and defends a view of medical ethics that is in effect libertarian.[9] These issues are complicated, but Engelhardt's moral skepticism reaches too far.

All of the aforementioned medical ethics models make valuable contributions to philosophy and the theory and practice of medical ethics. I present this work as one way to extend the moral tradition of moral pluralism by emphasizing the work of William David Ross and Beauchamp and Childress. I accept Ross's basic framework of *prima facie* principles that often conflict. Like Beauchamp and Childress, I accept the revisability of our moral concepts, but I depart from Ross, Beauchamp, and Childress in significant ways. I think many of our moral concepts are less fruitful than often realized, and the need to revise our views is a pressing need. I take the concept of incommensurability seriously and view much of the moral life as a constructive process. I realize that neither Ross nor Beauchamp and Childress would agree with some of my key concepts.

With the exception of Engelhardt, American medical ethicists virtually always assume that value conflicts involve commensurable alternatives. Conversely, many moral philosophers argue that in some cases, we have no compelling way to conclude which value in a conflict deserves priority.[10] In chapter three I show how we can understand the efficacy and limitations of morality by exploring the concept of incommensurability and the weighing metaphor.

If we take the weighing metaphor seriously then we have reason to be confident about the justification of some of our moral judgments, thereby overcoming the extreme skepticism of Engelhardt. The weighing metaphor suggests we are limited in making moral judgments, but does not adequately shed light on evaluating projects such as xenotransplantation and stem cell research. After all, many morally relevant consequences of our actions depend upon further human interventions and constitute a cluster of uncertainties and decisions that are different from evaluating the morality of a single action. Such projects do not lend themselves to moral discovery in the way of many moral decisions. This is why the past or present failure of an organ retrieval strategy such as xenotransplantation or the unproven success of other strategies such as stem cell research does not suffice as a reason to abandon that strategy. Greater resources, more intense efforts, and luck may finally lead to good results. These moral limitations mean that we do not always have the wherewithal to adequately compare our options; some options are incommensurable in fact even if not incommensurable in principle.

Some scholars believe the incommensurability of values confounds moral decision-making, but I indicate in Part Two and clarify in Part Three that we can make justified moral decision even if incommensurability is a widespread phenomenon.[11] These conclusions help explain the moral limitations of all people and serve as a springboard for emphasizing the good that we can accomplish amidst many uncertainties. With these philosophical considerations in mind, I illustrate my view of constructive pluralism by exploring the ethics of different organ retrieval strategies.

I begin an analysis of organ retrieval strategies by presenting evidence that organ transplants prove to be valuable for many patients. In chapter four, I summarize the literature on the quality of life for those who receive heart, liver, or kidney transplants. Although quality of life studies suffer from philosophical and methodological difficulties, evidence justifies the conclusion that organ transplants are valuable for many patients. The success of transplantation does not justify all organ retrieval practices and proposals, but it shows that failing to perform transplants on those patients who could benefit results in the premature loss of qualitatively meaningful lives. Transplantation has obvious moral value. Whether the success of transplantation justifies neglecting or violating other values in our quest for organs remains debatable.

In chapters five through nine, I examine different organ retrieval strategies. I do not examine all of the details, but my analysis reveals noteworthy conflicts and the potential moral losses resulting from these conflicts. These chapters also show that the organ retrieval literature underappreciates the ethical challenges and the possible adjustments we can make to develop a sound approach to the problem of premature organ failure.

In chapter five, I consider the ethics of routine retrieval, presumed consent, and familial consent. Routine retrieval amounts to taking organs without consent from those declared dead. Presumed consent means that we would assume decedents wished to donate unless they previously indicated otherwise. Familial consent provides a potential organ donor's family with the option to permit or nullify organ retrieval. Considering routine retrieval, presumed consent, and familial consent leads us to question whether we can wrong the dead by transgressing their prior wishes. Although I agree with many leading philosophers and medical ethicists who contend that dead persons deserve moral respect, difficulties remain as to how post-persons deserve present and future moral concern within influential views regarding necessary conditions for possessing moral status.

The apparent conflict between honoring the former wishes of the dead who did not want to donate and extending life for those awaiting transplantation results in a negative aftermath no matter what we do. Conflicts also arise when dead persons did wish to donate, but their family overrides their former wishes. Either we allow some transplant patients to die that we could have saved, or we potentially violate the former wishes of the dead, disturb many living persons' moral sensibilities, and risk discrediting the retrieval and transplant establishment.

In chapter six, I explain why the American medical and legal establishment changed the definition of death from the permanent cessation of the heart and lungs to the permanent cessation of the whole brain. We have learned that persons declared dead in accordance with the whole brain definition can still exhibit brain activity and produce hormones, apparent evidence of brain function. Consequently, some scholars defend returning to the cardiopulmonary definition.[12] Others advocate a higher brain definition in which physicians would declare death if and only if persons permanently lose consciousness.[13] Some higher brain defenders base their view on the permanent loss of personal identity in terms of being a unique person.[14]

These alternative definitions of death affect organ retrieval and transplantation differently. The whole brain definition allows for the preservation of a decedent's organs through artificial ventilation, but it prevents us from taking organs from other potential sources such as persistently vegetative patients. Acting based on the cardiopulmonary definition risks that organs might not receive enough blood and oxygen before retrieval thereby damaging the organs. Implementing the higher brain definition might lead to the retrieval of the most organs, but it violates many persons' intuitions as to what constitutes death. Persons who have permanently lost consciousness or other essential personal traits may still exhibit life signs such as spontaneous breathing. Again, the position likely to permit the retrieval of the most organs stretches credulity and risks diminishing the credibility and authority of the transplant community.

In chapter seven, I discuss whether selling organs is morally permissible. Transplant teams could retrieve organs once the seller dies, or, in cases involving a kidney, lung, or liver lobe, while the seller is alive. Financial incentives would increase the supply of transplantable organs, but risk exploiting the poor and treating persons as mere commodities. The selling of organs can take many forms ranging from compensating family members of organ sellers for funeral expenses to allowing financially destitute individuals to sell a kidney that will not substantially improve their standard of living. An ethical analysis of organ selling will need to explore the particulars of the system proposed and whether the system applies to living sellers, dead sellers, or both. We must also consider why selling organs has received more opposition than the selling of other bodily parts such as eggs, sperm, blood, or even hair.

In chapter eight, I discuss the ethics of animal transplants, or xenotransplants, the transplantation of organs and tissues of an individual of one species into a member of another species. Advocates of xenotransplants have chosen pigs to provide organs for humans for three reasons: the size of their organs, sows give birth to several piglets each year, and the piglets grow quickly.[15] Given the success of xenotransplants, many persons would have their lives extended. Transplanting pig organs into humans conflicts with the value of pigs' lives and risks spreading diseases to transplant recipients and to third parties. Xenotransplantation raises issues about animals' rights and welfare and the community's health versus the needs of individual patients.

In chapter nine, I discuss the ethics of promising new research with stem cells, the master cells that can develop into different tissues. In the future, we may be able to grow an unlimited supply of organs within laboratories. Stem cell research is controversial, though, because researchers take the cells from infertility clinics' leftover embryos and from aborted fetuses. Even if we support women's right to abortion and believe that embryos do not warrant the same level of moral consideration as infants, children, and adults, we still need to determine whether embryos and fetuses deserve any moral respect. If they do, then we must assess what this entails for research aimed at helping a variety of patients, including those with failing organs. Whether taking stem cells from living adult donors holds as much medical promise as using embryonic stem cells is also debatable.

Having discussed major residue-producing conflicts in the quest for transplantable organs, in chapter ten I discuss an alleged form of residue deemed the regulative principle: the requirement to avoid conflicts or dilemmas.[16] Even if we reject the idea that dilemmas exist in the previously defined sense, the regulative principle invites us to consider whether we ought to avoid all or many residue-producing conflicts. I argue that we should not attempt to avoid all residue-producing conflicts, but the regulative principle reminds us that avoiding some conflicts plays a crucial part in making a better world. An obvious application to organ retrieval is that preventing organ failure would circumvent many conflicts, a surprising gap in the literature on the ethics of organ retrieval and transplantation. I take the regulative principle further by arguing that even though we should not avoid all conflicts, values at stake in a conflict still guide us in terms of indicating appropriate attitudinal and behavioral responses by giving us reason to make adjustments for values that go unrealized or transgressed.

An emended version of the regulative principle has an interesting application to organ retrieval because we can manipulate the number of organs retrieved in many ways by making conceptual, psychological, social, legal, medical, institutional, or technological adjustments. These adjustments illustrate the dynamic nature of organ retrieval. The multitude of possible adjustments leads us to evaluate a cluster of organ retrieval strategies and to compare the moral value of these combinations of strategies. But how are we to compare the value of alternatives? In addition, since I argue that some alternatives are incommensurable, what are we to do?

In chapter eleven, I clarify what I mean by constructive pluralism. As Beauchamp and Childress suggest, I explore the revisions needed with regard to our concepts, practices, and institutions. Like Engelhardt, I emphasize the problem with comparing our options. I also show what the recognition of incommensurable alternatives suggests for making revisions to achieve a valuable life. Despite counterintuitive inclinations, we can make rational comparisons even in the midst of widespread incommensurability. I believe we have often been looking at ethics and medical ethics in the wrong light by focusing on making moral discoveries instead of on building a valuable life with limited moral resources. This is not to establish a strict dichotomy between discovering and building, but to show how too much emphasis on finding moral discoveries leads to inadequate moral thinking.

By *constructive* pluralism, I am not placing this work within the tradition known as social constructivism. Any similarities thereof are coincidental. I use "constructive" to emphasize the continual and often difficult process of doing good works. My account is constructive in the sense that making good things happen by our actions and by articulating and reassessing our conceptualization of values takes a central role in the moral life. This construction includes reevaluations of traditional values in terms of their content and application. I also emphasize the broader social context of ethical decisions regarding organ retrieval and the many ways available to us in addressing the problem of premature organ failure. That is, I elaborate on the many adjustments available to us in the quest to retrieve more organs. The ongoing conceptual, technological, medical, legal, social, psychological, institutional, and ethical adjustments necessary for addressing conflict and developing a good life constitutes a constructive process.

My response is pluralistic in the sense of what is good and of what is right. Many values such as respect for persons, happiness, self-achievement, growth of knowledge, friendship, and love constitute morally relevant features of moral decision-making. As the foregoing remarks indicate, these values create conflicts that generate losses, residue, and indeterminacy. Regarding right action, many actions are morally acceptable, even given the contextual details. Contra many accounts of moral pluralism, contextual details cannot always or most always indicate single right answers to moral questions regarding how a conflict should be resolved.[17] I also argue for the unconventional thesis that some moral problems have no single best response, even apart from symmetrical cases of conflicts involving equal values. This view stands in stark contrast to conventional medical ethics in which medical ethicists write as if their deliberations on issues should find a single right answer once they account for the relevant facts, values, and probabilities.

In turn, constructive pluralism changes the way we view conflicts, losses, and residue. Conflicts may result from the way we conceptualize our values and morally relevant concepts, not only the reality of the moral life. Inadequate concepts may be at the root of the frustratingly difficult challenge of defining death and in determining which entities deserve moral respect. Given incommensurable alternatives and the importance of continuous interventions in constructing a better world, the moral losses and residue we face become more conditional and fluid than usually conceived. That is, many of our residual requirements and recommendations depend on other decisions, efforts, and luck. In the final analysis, this means that medical ethics must address an open-ended world. We can make the world morally appropriate in different ways assuming that we make necessary adjustments to accommodate previous choices.

What counts as morally appropriate thought and behavior is limited. Any justifiable moral decision must include the attempt to realize values and include strategies to limit the losses of unrealized or transgressed values. For this reason, constructive pluralism does not open the moral floodgates regarding what should count as ethical conduct. Persons have no justification for being indifferent to or complacent about the fallout of their decisions, even good decisions. When values do not issue unique directives, they still guide action by indicating a range of permissible actions and by providing the basis to make an adjustment to avoid or limit our moral losses or to adopt an appropri-

ate attitude regarding our choices and their consequences. Constructive pluralism is an interpretation of the moral life as elastic but with boundaries.

In the end, I summarize my findings and attempt to deflect worries about
viewing all of the moral life as a constructive process instead of viewing the
moral life as a process of attempting to make moral discoveries. I do think
moral discoveries are a significant part of life. After all, I assume we can discover moral conflicts; many conflicts are a part of the world, not just our concepts. Second, I believe questions about what to do about contemporary moral
problems sometimes have discoverable answers, even unique answers. Third,
I try to show that we can have a robust morality in the sense that moral values
can be response guiding even without indicating unique resolutions to difficult conflicts. Reflection discovers that some moral conflicts lend themselves
to a plurality of justifiable responses and that we have reason to make adjustments for unrealized or transgressed values.

In conclusion, the moral approach to the problem of people suffering
from congenital or premature organ failure is largely a constructive process
whereby we embark on some justifiable strategies that realize values, make
adjustments to alleviate the fallout of conflicts, and prevent some conflicts. I
mean this as both an interpretation of our past and current actions and practices and as an invitation to become more aware of our multiple opportunities
to lead moral, but imperfect lives as individuals, members of nations, and as
members of a global community. Which paths we should take remains puzzling at times, but some strategies cannot be justified. We can defend decisions involving conflicts given that we are committed to making morally required or reasonable adjustments. The question becomes, how malleable are
we as individuals, nations, and a global community?

Although this work leaves many issues unresolved, I hope to have contributed to the philosophical and bioethical literature in the following ways. I
systematically consider the ramifications of residue-producing conflicts for
organ transplantation. Many moral philosophers mention moral residue, but it
has not received detailed attention. While most medical ethicists concentrate
on applying or criticizing Beauchamp and Childress's four-principle model, I
focus on illustrating their views on our moral limits and the need to make revisions within a moral belief system. I address the philosophical literature by
analyzing the regulative principle and defending the thesis that we should not
avoid all conflicts but that values guide our attitudes and actions by indicating
a range of justifiable decisions and adjustments we may make in response to
moral losses. I show that widespread incommensurability does not necessarily
undermine good decision-making. I also critically discuss the literature on
whether we can wrong the dead, defining death, selling organs, xenotransplantation, and stem cells. This work invites new and vigorous discussion of
value conflicts, residue, pluralism, organ retrieval strategies, and the prevention of premature or congenital organ failure.

Part One

A PHILOSOPHICAL FRAMEWORK

One

DILEMMAS, CONFLICTS, AND RESIDUE

> It is sometimes hard, however, to judge what (goods) should be chosen
> at the price of what (evils), and what (evils) should be endured as the
> price of what (goods). And it is even harder to abide by our judgment,
> since the results we expect (when we endure) are usually painful, and the
> actions we are compelled (to endure, when we choose) are usually
> shameful. That is why those who have been compelled or not compelled
> receive praise and blame.[1]

In William Styron's stunning novel, *Sophie's Choice*, the Nazi invasion of Po-
land forces many Poles, including Sophie and her son and daughter, to im-
prisonment at Auschwitz.[2] There a Nazi officer notices Sophie's beauty, and
he abruptly tells her that he wants to go to bed with her. He also tells her that
he knows she is a "Polack," and he asks her whether she is a "filthy commu-
nist." Struck with terror, Sophie attempts to appease him by informing him in
German that she and her children are Polish, not Jewish, and that she is a
Christian. As if he prepared for such a moment, he rhetorically asks Sophie
whether Jesus Christ said, "Suffer the little children to come unto Me." He
then demands that Sophie choose between the lives of her children. She
screams that she cannot make that choice, but he orders her to choose or both
children will die. Although she never articulates her reason, she tells him to
take her daughter, a choice that plagues her with suffocating guilt.

Some moral philosophers characterize Sophie's choice as the paradig-
matic dilemma, a situation wherein she faces two moral requirements that she
is unable to fulfill.[3] According to these dilemma defenders, Sophie has a
moral requirement to save her son and a moral requirement to save her daughter, even though she cannot do both. This conception of dilemma generates
controversy because the failure to act on a moral requirement suggests
wrongdoing and blameworthiness. The Nazi officer's actions warrant con-
demnation, but the moral merits of Sophie's choice remains contentious.

Surprisingly, a fair number of prominent moral philosophers deny the
possibility of dilemmas in the sense of circumstances in which persons have
more moral requirements than they can possibly fulfill.[4] Philosophers inclined
to exonerate Sophie, for instance, can acknowledge the tragic proportions of
her predicament, but deny she faces conflicting moral requirements. To the
minds of these dilemma opponents, it only appears that Sophie faces two incompatible requirements. Again, they can recognize the tragic conditions, but
claim Sophie (and anyone else for that matter) can have at most one require-

ment for each choice. On this view, she has a requirement to save one of her children, but it does not matter morally which one she chooses. The reason for this conclusion is that Sophie's options are symmetrical: her children possess equal moral value, and sacrificing one for the sake of the other is better than allowing both to die. The moral dimensions of Sophie's choice invite endless debate. In this book, I will focus on another facet of difficult, even tragic, moral choices, the moral losses and residue of decisions that are understandable, justified, or even optimal given the circumstances.

Sophie's choice demonstrates that, no matter what we do, some decisions will leave moral residue in the form of guilt, regret, or remorse, requirements to repair the harm done, and requirements to avoid such conflicts. Even if Sophie does not face a dilemma strictly speaking, she faces a horrible conflict. Both defenders and opponents of dilemmas agree that many conflicts leave us with moral residue. All parties to the debate over the existence of dilemmas assume the existence of residue-producing conflicts.

Interestingly, in many cases both defenders and opponents of dilemmas seek to exonerate persons trapped in difficult conflicts while accounting for all forms of moral residue. I call this effort the accomodationist project. The accomodationist project creates conceptual problems because dilemma defenders have difficulty exonerating persons trapped in dilemmas, whereas dilemma opponents have difficulty accounting for all forms of residue.

Beginning with a clarification of terms such as "dilemma," "conflict," "value," and "residue," I then explore the concept of residue by evaluating the accommodationist project. This exploration includes a discussion of appraising the character of persons trapped in alleged dilemmas and conflicts and of the moral requirements and recommendations generated by alleged dilemmas and conflicts. I present the challenges of the accommodationist project, but ultimately develop a practical position in which we can acknowledge residue-producing conflicts without taking a side in the dilemma debate. This analysis paves the way for exploring the moral import of residue-producing conflicts in the quest to retrieve or create more organs that are transplantable.

1. Terminology

I use the term "dilemma" for situations involving incompatible moral requirements: circumstances where a person or group faces a requirement to do A, a requirement to do B, and yet the person cannot accomplish A and B. Since we infrequently know whether actions are impossible to perform together or merely unlikely, another conception of dilemma incorporates human limitations about knowing the future, even the near future. That is, a person trapped in an alleged dilemma would believe that A and B cannot both be done; the person's belief would be justified, but true or false. Perhaps Sophie could have found a way to save both of her children, but it did not appear as though she could. At any rate, the persons trapped in the apparent dilemmas discussed in this chapter are justified in thinking their options are limited to the choices specified in the description of the alleged dilemma. As this book unfolds, thinking about our alternatives regarding retrieving and creating organs is crucial. Before proceeding to other terms, we should note one more point about the meaning of "dilemma."

Patricia Greenspan distinguishes between positive and negative dilemmas.[5] Positive dilemmas involve choices between two mutually exclusive and jointly exhaustive actions a person is required to perform; negative dilemmas mean that a person must choose between forbidden actions. The previous description of Sophie's choice as one between two requirements counts as a positive dilemma. Greenspan believes she complicates Sophie's choice even further by recasting it as a situation where the dictates of morality forbid her from sacrificing her son, forbid her from sacrificing her daughter, and forbid her from allowing both of them to die.[6] On this account, Sophie faces a negative dilemma. Greenspan believes that, all other things remaining equal, negative dilemmas damage a person's character more so than positive dilemmas. In either case, the existence of dilemmas remains contentious because they leave persons without any way to do all that morality requires or forbids.

In contrast to supposed dilemmas, conflicts consist of values that provide the basis for only one requirement or none at all: a valuable action can be permissible or recommended instead of required. A positive conflict means that possible actions A and B are recommended for realizing something morally valuable, but doing both A and B is improbable or impossible. One but not both of the acts may be required. A negative conflict means reasons exist for avoiding possible actions C and D, but avoiding both C and D is unlikely or impossible. Similarly, morality forbids one but not both of the possible actions. We can also imagine cases where a person is supposed to refrain from actions, but refraining from those actions is worse than performing one of them. Sophie's choice apparently fits this situation.

Many conflicts stemming from organ retrieval and transplantation practices and proposals involve conflicting possible actions that will probably lead to something good and bad or permit something good and bad. The moral import of actions pertaining to organ retrieval and transplantation is often mixed. Xenotransplants, for example, offer hope to future patients, but cause the death of animals and risk spreading diseases to xenotransplant recipients and to third parties. On the other hand, refraining from xenotransplant research may result in the loss of more human lives.

Although courses of action can be valuable for many reasons (prudential, moral, aesthetic, and epistemological), I will focus on clashes between possible actions that have moral value. Actions are morally valuable when they either consist of or lead to intrinsic values—goods appropriately valued for their own sake.

Philosophers do not always agree on the number or types of intrinsic values. Jeremy Bentham notoriously equated value with pleasure, holding that pleasure is a single sort of experience with varying degrees.[7] Immanuel Kant believed all moral value amounts to respect for persons where "persons" means rational agents capable of legislating his or her behavior.[8] Others take a pluralist approach. William David Ross counted pleasure, knowledge, justice, and virtuous disposition as intrinsically valuable.[9] Charles Taylor includes personal integrity, agape, liberation, rationality, and comfort on his list.[10] Michael Stocker mentions sensual pleasure, wisdom, and honor as types of values.[11] Others subdivide values such as pleasure and individual liberty. The pleasure from drinking beer, smelling roses, and having sexual intercourse are phenomenologically different: our subjective experience registers qualitative distinctions among pleasures.[12] Isaiah Berlin distinguishes between negative and positive liberty, the value of being free from harm and the interference of others appears different from the freedom to embark on meaningful projects.[13]

Living well requires the attainment of intrinsic values and the avoidance of something bad as well. Candidates for negative moral values, call them disvalues, include harm, pain, coercion, ignorance, foolishness, hate, a lack of respect for persons, and so forth.

I see no way to determine an exhaustive list of intrinsic values and disvalues. Reflection shows that the moral life involves a plurality of values. A sense of peace differs from gourmet pleasures; emotional suffering differs from physical pain. Pain can be throbbing, piercing, or burning. As we will see, our list of intrinsic values and disvalues impacts the way we view different proposals to retrieve or create transplantable organs.

The plurality of values and disvalues forms the basis of constructive pluralism in two significant ways. First, although a plurality of intrinsic values is not necessary or sufficient for conflicts, in this world, a plurality of intrinsic values and disvalues results in many conflicts. Second, the plurality of intrinsic values and disvalues is one reason for the incommensurability of some conflicts. We cannot always make justifiable judgments as to which value in a conflict deserves priority or which disvalue is worse. In turn, the incommensurability of values has an interesting and often overlooked connection to the plurality of right action, the view that some circumstances allow for more than one justified response.

For a possible action to provide moral reasons for its performance, the possible action must either contain or lead to some positive intrinsic value or avoid some disvalue. Again, there may be many non-moral reasons for permitting, recommending, requiring, or forbidding an action, but for the purposes of this book, I am interested in moral evaluations of performing or refraining from actions. Whenever I mention "conflict," "conflict of values," "conflicting values," or "value conflicts," I will be referring to instances where intrinsic moral values give us some reason to perform different actions or where disvalues provide reasons to avoid an action. Readers should understand that for better or worse, I have a broad view of the moral life.

Again, the debate over dilemmas concerns whether we can sometimes face conflicting requirements. I will use "requirement," though the use of "obligation" and "duty" are common throughout the literature. "Requirement" indicates in a strong binding sense a reason to perform an action or to adopt an attitude, a topic that will gain clarification. I will also refer to one type of residue—leftover requirements—as "residual requirements."

Moral losses can occur without the presence of conflicting values. We can and do act badly out of ignorance, moral weakness, and self interest, and much pain and suffering results from our intellectual and biological limits, not only from life's unkind and sometimes brutal conflicting impositions. Difficult or tragic choices that consist of or produce moral losses are painfully familiar. New to the philosophical literature is discussion of the moral implications of the moral losses of decisions that are understandable, justified, or even optimal in given circumstances. At times, I will refer to these losses as "aftermath," and "fallout." Moral losses from a choice between conflicting values may result in harmful or painful consequences or consist in transgressions of moral requirements or failures to act on recommendations that are intrinsically wrong, or both. This account, then, draws from consequentialist and deontological traditions.

Following Terrance McConnell, I will use "residue" to refer to the moral implications of the aftermath of conflicts or alleged dilemmas such as appropriate negative emotions, guilt, remorse, or regret, and residual requirements to make amends or explain oneself, and requirements to avoid future conflicts or dilemmas.[14] Scholars have also used "remainder" in place of "residue," but "residue" has been the term that most commentators utilize.[15] That said, I will turn to the substance of residue and the dilemma debate. For the purposes of this book, I focus on residual requirements and recommendations instead of on guilt, remorse, and regret, but I show in chapter ten that appropriate negative emotions are crucial for understanding conflicts and the guiding nature of morality. I will also focus on the requirement to avoid conflicts in chapter ten.

2. Moral Residue

The quotation from Aristotle beginning this chapter indicates an ancient understanding of the mixed results of responding to conflicts. The early twentieth-century philosopher Ross first explicated our contemporary understanding of residue, though I do not believe he coined the term. In Ross's words:

> When we think ourselves justified in breaking, and indeed morally obliged to break, a promise in order to relieve some one's distress, we do not for a moment cease to recognize a prima facie duty to keep our

promise, and this leads us to feel, not indeed shame or repentance, but certainly compunction, for behaving as we do; we recognize, further, that it is our duty to make up somehow to the promisee for the breaking of the promise.[16]

I use "requirement" instead of "duty" or "obligation," and I assume these terms are synonymous. Ross discusses conflicting *prima facie* duties to illustrate a conflict. Usually, "*prima facie*" means "at first appearance" or "on the surface." But this cannot be what Ross means. The mere appearance of conflicting duties does not indicate a real conflict that would result in the need to make amends. I agree with David Owen Brink who interprets Ross's use of "*prima facie*" as meaning that a *prima facie* evaluation provides a reason to perform an act in the absence of a conflicting *prima facie* evaluation.[17] The need to act in accordance with a *prima facie* evaluation does not vanish just because a person justifiably acts upon a different *prima facie* evaluation.

Ross means that the breaking of the promise violates a moral requirement. The moral violation provides reasons to feel compunction and provides the basis of a requirement to do something to make up for breaking the promise. The requirement to make amends is the moral residue.

More recently, Bernard Williams has been principally responsible for stimulating discussion on the implications of conflicts. Williams considers a case in which a man promises his father to support an identified charity after his father's death. After his father dies, the man lacks money to both support the charity and adequately provide for his children. In Williams's terms, the man faces a clash of obligations. Apparently, the man has an obligation to support the charity and an obligation to provide for his children, but, by hypothesis, cannot do both. A resolution would be easy if the man made the initial promise under the tacit assumption that fulfillment of supporting the charity did not interfere with significant matters like caring for his children. If that were the case, Williams believes the obligation to keep his promise would evaporate and leave no conflict at all.[18] Like Ross, Williams believes conflicting values can provide obligatory reasons for performing different actions; each action produces residue when not performed. In Williams's words:

> There are certainly two obligations in a real case of this kind, though one may outweigh the other. The one that outweighs has greater stringency, but the one that is outweighed also possesses some stringency, and this is expressed in what, by way of compensation, I may have to do for the parties who are disadvantaged by its being outweighed; whether I have merely to explain and apologise, or whether I have to engage further in some more substantial reparatory action.[19]

Unfortunately, Williams fails to clarify the sort of case to which he refers. I doubt that he is still referring to the case of the man who promised to assist the charity, even though the quoted passage is introduced a few lines after the presentation of that case since he calls the case relatively painless.[20] It makes no sense to call a case relatively painless when it may call for substantial reparations. Still, we can understand his point that neglecting the less stringent obligation creates residue in the form of a reason to make reparations.

3. Epistemology and Ontology of Dilemmas

Those unfamiliar with the debate over whether dilemmas exist may wonder why anyone, much less a group of intelligent, sensitive persons, could doubt the possibility of conflicting moral requirements. The indecision and emotional struggles we often experience when confronted with issues such as abortion, capital punishment, physician-assisted suicide, and the aforementioned conflicts with retrieving and transplanting organs suggest the reality of dilemmas and their frequency as well. Fortunately, understanding the difference between the ontological and epistemological dimensions of dilemmas clarifies the reason for the debate.

In many cases, defenders of dilemmas are not making an epistemological point; their point is ontological. That is, we find ourselves in dilemmas not merely because of limited knowledge about what we ought to do, but because life has made impossible moral demands on us. If dilemmas were strictly epistemological, then it would always remain possible that a sufficiently well informed person would know exactly what to do in each situation. In that case, dilemmas would be apparent but not real: apparent in the sense that only limited information stands in the way of always recognizing a single requirement or best response, or that different actions are equally justifiable.

The usual assumption has been that for each person in each circumstance many responses can be morally permissible, but, at most, only one action can be required. Defenders of dilemmas think that even fully informed individuals, even an omniscient person, could not always select a uniquely correct action for some situations. Dilemma defenders believe two incompatible actions may be required and equally stringent. In other cases, we may know that an option is more valuable than an alternative, but even the less stringent option may be required as well. Dilemmas do not only appear to be real because our information is limited. Dilemmas are part of reality. That is just the way of the world, an undesirable moral reality.

With a better understanding of the difference between the epistemological and ontological dimensions of alleged dilemmas, I will address the worries of dilemma opponents. Once we address the moral implications of alleged dilemmas, we will be in a better position to determine whether dilemmas exist. In turn, the consideration of consequences will help us understand the nature of residue and its relevance for understanding significant features of our moral lives such as those encountered when responding to persons who need a transplant.

4. Dilemmas and Deontic Logic

To understand the debate over dilemmas, it helps to discuss the basic principles of deontic logic; logic devoted to correct moral reasoning. Deontic logic is a type of logic devoted to correct inferences regarding what is required and what is permissible. According to standard deontic logic, moral dilemmas are impossible, because assuming that dilemmas exist leads to a contradiction. Although this information is technical, it helps clarify the debates. In chapter three, we find that some medical ethicists raise the issue of disagreement over correct moral inferences. Debates over dilemmas and deontic logic contributed to many issues about the action guiding nature of morality and whether we ought to avoid conflict.

Consider the following standard formal interpretation of dilemmas as applied to Sophie's choice:

Let A = Sophie saves her son.
Let B = Sophie saves her daughter.
Let C = It is possible that . . .
Let R = It is required that . . .
Let P = It is permitted that . . .
Let & = and
Let ~ = not
Let ⊃ = if . . . then; so, A ⊃ B means "if A, then B."
(P1) (R)A & (R)B
(P2) ~(C)(A & B)

Premises (P1) and (P2) represent the standard interpretation of a dilemma. Coupling these premises with the closure principle, ((R)B & ~(C)(A & B)) ⊃ (R)~A, yields (R)~A. Premise (P1) posits (R)A, so we have (R)A & (R)~A. Likewise, since the dilemma requires Sophie to perform A as well, we can derive (R)B & (R)~B. The "ought" implies "permissible" principle states that if A is morally required, A is permissible. The principle is formalized as (R)A ⊃ ~(P)~A. The logical rule called transposition allows us to then derive ~((R)A & (R)~A). Another way of putting this point is that (P)A ⊃ ~(R)~A, and ~((R)A & (R)~A). In a few steps we can show how positing dilemmas leads to a contradiction: ((R)A & (R)~A) & ~((R)A & (R)~A).

We can derive other contradictions as well. The "ought" implies "can" principle claims that if we ought to perform an action, then we are capable of performing that action. Assuming a strong sense of "ought," logicians formalize the principle as (R)A ⊃ (C)A. We have already learned that (R)A & (R)~A can be derived from the formalized interpretation of dilemmas. The agglomeration principle states that if we ought to do A and we ought to do B, then we ought to do A and B. Agglomeration is formalized as (R)A & (R)~A ⊃ (R)(A & ~A). By applying the "ought" implies "can" principle we can derive (C)(A & ~A). This shows that the conjunction of agglomeration and "ought" implies "can" with the standard interpretation of dilemmas leads to another contradiction. These contradictions indicate either that dilemmas do not exist or that we need to abandon or revise standard deontic logic. Interestingly, Brink is the only person I know of who defends some principles of deontic logic in the context of the debate over dilemmas.[21] Some scholars state that we should reject deontic logic if it conflicts with belief in dilemmas.[22]

As an alternative to characterizing Sophie's choice and other alleged dilemmas as incompatible requirements, others suggest interpreting such situations as a disjunctive requirement, a requirement to perform one option.[23] So, Sophie has a requirement to save one of her children. Regarding alleged dilemmas as disjunctive requirements makes it difficult to explain how such predicaments leave persons facing the decision with reasons to compensate or make amends to someone, to explain him or herself, or adopt a regretful attitude. Sophie's situation, for example, does not parallel situations involving an obvious disjunctive requirement.

Suppose a surgeon who received financial aid to pay for medical school must meet a condition of the financial aid contract by treating disadvantaged patients in some remote area. The surgeon has, say, a disjunctive requirement to serve those in community *A*, community *B*, or community *C*. To the surprise of cynics, the surgeon happily serves the needs of one remote community. In this case, the surgeon does not owe compensation, an apology, or an explanation to the people of the communities not chosen. Nor should the surgeon feel guilty for not selecting the other communities. This example shows a distinction between some disjunctive requirements and some alleged dilemmas. As previous examples show, the distinction is not merely the severity of the consequences. The difference is the relationship between the person in the predicament with respect to the available options. This example also shows that a conflict of values does not necessarily create residue for the person facing the conflict. The needs of the other communities do not disappear. For this reason, we should still describe the surgeon's choice as a conflict on the basis that others will have moral reason to meet the needs of those communities where the surgeon does not choose to serve.

5. Guilt, Regret, and Remorse

Part of the debate over dilemmas pertains to the moral psychological consequences of facing incompatible moral requirements. In the argument from guilt, regret, and remorse, dilemma defenders can argue for situations in which agents will appropriately feel moral guilt, regret, or remorse only if they have done something wrong. Persons can appropriately feel moral guilt, regret, or remorse regardless of what they do. It follows, then, that in some situations persons act wrongly no matter what they do. Persons perform a wrong action only if they violate a moral requirement. In some situations persons necessarily violate a moral requirement based on the circumstances instead of moral weakness; such traps constitute a dilemma.

In this spirit, Thomas Nagel claims dilemmas present, "us with situations in which there is no honorable or moral course for a man to take, no course free of guilt and responsibility for evil."[24] Similarly, Bas C. van Fraassen characterizes the existentialist's hero as one, "who does not fail to act upon his ideals, and does not rationalize away his dirty hands."[25] Alan Harry Donagan qualifies this point by saying that persons are only necessarily blameworthy for what they do in a dilemma, if they brought about that dilemma through previous wrongdoing.[26] Nagel and van Fraassen differ from many commentators in that they do not defend some version of the accomodationist project.

Defenders of dilemmas have not seriously considered the implications of dilemmas for medical ethics, but Greenspan discusses a case where a doctor must choose between two transplant candidates who both meet medical criteria for a successful transplantation.[27] According to Greenspan, the doctor would not be guilty of wrongdoing as long as the doctor attempts to save one patient. She distinguishes positive and negative dilemmas. The doctor's case involves exclusive requirements, but the requirement to save one patient disappears, once the doctor decides which patient to save. In Greenspan's mind, the doctor's case differs from Sophie's choice because the doctor does not select one patient to die so another may live. In contrast, Sophie gives her son an opportunity to live only by sacrificing her daughter.

I agree with Greenspan that the doctor is not guilty of wrongdoing in a case where the doctor must choose between patients to save who could equally benefit from a transplant. I am not convinced of a relevant difference between Sophie's choice interpreted as a case of exclusive requirements to save her children, or as exhaustive prohibitions not to sacrifice her children. My hesitation to accept Greenspan's position revolves around the familiar distinction between taking an action that leads to a person's death and failing to prevent a person's death. We know this distinction as doing versus allowing or killing versus letting die.

Over the years, I have found that I have inconsistent intuitions regarding the killing-letting die distinction. In some cases it appears that allowing a person to die is just as bad as killing that person; in other cases killing appears worse. This may indicate that I am inconsistent, the distinction is suspect, or both. No matter the truth about the moral significance of the killing-letting die distinction, we have other reasons to consider in an attempt to exonerate Sophie, doctors who must choose among transplant candidates, and persons who may find themselves in circumstances where they must choose between the lives of their children.

6. Autonomy and Wrongdoing

Thomas Hill rejects the view that dilemmas exist based on the Kantian autonomy principle, the principle stating that persons are morally responsible in the circumstances if and only if they can fulfill their moral requirements in those circumstances for the sake of their requirements.[28] A commitment to the principle of autonomy entails that persons have done no wrong where they had no choice. Persons should not feel like they have done wrong for failing to do good or from preventing evil whenever they could not have done so. Since dilemmas require agents to do what is impossible, agents trapped in dilemmas cannot freely act on all of their moral requirements. A commitment to dilemmas appears to violate the autonomy principle.

In Hill's view, we should evaluate wrongness and blameworthiness in terms of a person's knowledge, opportunities, and abilities in specified contexts. The point of morality, he claims, is to offer guidance for all deliberative agents, even those guilty of landing themselves into further moral conflicts.[29] He dismisses dilemmas on the grounds that they condemn agents, even well intentioned agents, who do as well as circumstances allow. Hill can easily exonerate members of transplant teams who cannot help all patients in need. For the same reason, he can exonerate Sophie as well.

The autonomy issue is complicated, because persons caught in alleged dilemmas are free to act on each of the options. Sophie was free to tell the Nazi to save her son, free to tell the Nazi to save her daughter, and free to refrain from sacrificing either child. Exonerating agents such as Sophie based on the autonomy principle requires us to claim that to be autonomous in a given circumstance we must be free to perform all of our requirements in that case. This move begs the question against dilemma defenders. As we have seen, many philosophers believe that a person might have a requirement to perform an action that she cannot do.

The issue of inevitable wrongdoing does not necessarily divide defenders of dilemmas from their opponents. Recall that many contributors to the dilemmas debate are accomodationists in that they seek to account for residue while exonerating persons who choose well or what is best in conflicting circumstances. Walter Sinnott-Armstrong, a defender of dilemmas, absolves agents in dilemmas as long as they choose to fulfill one requirement.[30] To sort through the debate we must determine when appraisals of wrongdoing are appropriate and when appropriate guilt indicates wrongdoing.

7. Survivor's Guilt

An obvious objection to the contention that appropriate guilt always indicates wrongdoing is that survivors of disasters often feel guilty when others died. I know of a man who feels guilty for being alive, because many of his friends died from AIDS. Survivors often feel that they are no more deserving of life than those who died, but this does not mean that they feel morally responsible for those deaths. They know that they were not responsible. Assuming survivor's guilt is sometimes appropriate, appropriate guilt does not necessarily indicate wrongdoing. Showing that a person might necessarily do something for which guilt would be appropriate does not straightforwardly establish the presence of a dilemma.

Given survivor's guilt, dilemma defenders can distinguish types of guilt. They could amend their position to say persons will appropriately experience some type of guilt no matter what they do. This places pressure on dilemma defenders to determine whether a person feels a special type of guilt, or some other negative emotion that might be mistaken for this type of guilt. Without this emotion-identifying ability, parties to the dilemma debate will have recourse to disagree on the emotions a person may appropriately experience after making difficult moral choices. How can we determine people's emotions in tough moral circumstances? How can the persons themselves sort out their emotions?

8. The Nature of Emotion

In ordinary discourse, we commonly equate emotions with feelings or sensations. Frithjof Bergmann offers a simple but compelling view distinguishing emotions from physical sensations. While physical sensations are few, pleasures, pains, sensations of heat and coolness, emotions are many: love, admiration, respect, hatred, anger, disappointment, joy, surprise, envy, sadness, contentment, regret, and guilt for example.[31] Thus, emotions cannot be identical to sensations. Otherwise, there would be an equal number of sensations and emotions. Even if we can identify more types of sensations, the point still stands, because we can identify even more emotions than those just mentioned. What then constitutes an emotion? In addition to sensations, behavior and cognitive judgments constitute emotions.

Bergmann instructs us that when we are determining whether we are experiencing shame or embarrassment, a sensation does not inform us as to what we are experiencing. Instead, we attempt to determine whether we feel responsible for the actions giving rise to the experience broadly conceived. A cognitive judgment, in part, constitutes the emotion. He adds that we cannot reasonably claim to feel timid, loving, or compassionate without appeal to our behavior. The behavioral component helps explain why a person can have an emotion without the person knowing about it. A person can sincerely deny being jealous while the person's behavior suggests otherwise.[32] I accept Bergmann's view that emotions consist of sensations, cognitive judgments, and behavior. Significant for our purposes, participants in the debate over dilemmas accept the view that cognitive judgments are relevant to determining whether a person experiences guilt, remorse, regret, or sadness.

McConnell takes dilemma defenders to task regarding what agents who have allegedly faced dilemmas actually experience in the way of negative emotions. McConnell attacks the argument from guilt and remorse on two grounds. He concedes that in some situations persons ought to experience some negative emotion no matter what they do, but this emotion may not be guilt or remorse. He suggests that they experience regret. He adds that regret does not necessarily signal a sense of wrongdoing. As an example, he notes that a parent may appropriately regret punishing his child even when the parent acts justifiably. He also says a person may appropriately feel regret over, "the damage that a recent fire has caused to my neighbor's house, the pain that severe birth defects cause in infants, and the suffering experienced by a starving animal in the wilderness."[33] Similarly, we can regret or feel sad about animals that die to provide a source of xenotransplants, or about transplant candidates who die, in part, as a result from our decision to reject the routine retrieval of organs or presumed consent, even though we might feel justified in our decisions affecting the number of organs available for transplantation.

According to McConnell, we can distinguish regret from remorse and guilt on cognitive grounds. He suggests that the phenomenology of regret, remorse, and guilt, our subjective experience of them, may be indistinguishable, especially since each emotion may vary in intensity. For him, the cognitive component distinguishes negative emotions: remorse and guilt include the belief that one has acted wrongly, regret does not.[34]

If we accept McConnell's view of regret, remorse, and guilt, we must agree with him that dilemma defenders beg the question in saying some situations appropriately lead to remorse or guilt no matter what a person does or refrains from doing.[35]

To strengthen his case, McConnell adds that even appropriate remorse does not entail wrongdoing. Presumably, he would make the same claim about guilt. He has us imagine a person who, without fault, kills a child in an auto accident.[36] We are to suppose that the driver was alert and practicing the relevant safety measures at the time of the tragedy. At one level, McConnell tells us the person should not feel guilty in the sense of claiming wrongdoing.

Yet, the person may appropriately feel guilty or remorseful in the sense of recognizing one's causal connection to the misfortune.[37] A carefully constructed argument showing that a person appropriately feels guilt other than survivors' guilt does not prove wrongdoing. A circumstance wherein a person ought to feel guilty no matter how the person acts does not establish the presence of a dilemma.

Understandably, McConnell attempts to show that even the demonstration that a person should experience remorse or guilt regardless of what the person does in a situation does not entail the person acted wrongly. He is trying to show that a vast array of appropriate negative emotions in response to alleged dilemmas does not actually establish the presence of a dilemma. In this case, recognizing our causal contribution to a tragedy is different from believing that we acted wrongly. Maybe McConnell is right about this, but we must wonder whether McConnell is stipulating instead of arguing that a self-judgment of wrongdoing is what separates regret from guilt and remorse.

Sinnott-Armstrong, a dilemma defender, argues in much the same way. He has us suppose a situation where an injury to a child requires a hospital visit.[38] The mother recognizes her child's need for medical attention, but construction materials block her driveway. The only way she can get her daughter to the hospital is by driving through one yard on either side of her, but both yards have beautiful flower gardens in the way. Although she behaves correctly by plowing through one of her neighbor's gardens to care for her daughter, Sinnott-Armstrong believes the woman appropriately feels remorse about destroying her neighbor's flowers. He recognizes that others will claim she only feels regret, but he believes that to argue about what she actually feels amounts to a semantic quibble. If we think calling her remorseful implies that she transgressed an overriding requirement (a requirement that has priority over any conflicting requirement), or that she should be judged as a bad person, then she could not be appropriately remorseful. If we mean she understands that had her daughter not needed a hospital visit, it would have been wrong for her to drive through the flowers, then we should consider her remorseful. He states that what the agent feels is not the regret of the aesthete who notices the ravaged garden. He adds that the agent is not morally excused, because she could have driven over the other person's drive way.

The similarities between McConnell and Sinnott-Armstrong go further. Remember that McConnell argues against dilemmas, while Sinnott-Armstrong defends them. Both believe that agents can be appropriately remorseful without believing that they acted wrongly and when they have not acted wrongly. Both philosophers also believe that in alleged dilemmas third parties should not necessarily judge them as a bad person or as having acted badly or wrongly. Perhaps, though, Bergmann's inclusion of behavior in the identification of emotions will help resolve the debate.

Let us return to Sophie's predicament. If we consider Sophie's behavior after the Nazis murder her daughter, probably murder her son, and abuse her, Sophie experienced many negative emotions. The question is how do we know which behaviors would distinguish one negative emotion from another? Perhaps some philosophers, psychologists, or other mental health professionals have a method for individuating emotions. Judging by the literature on dilemmas, philosophers have not unequivocally delineated which emotions individuals experience or should experience when faced with dilemmas. We can stipulate the character of an emotion, but to individuate emotions we would have to evaluate the definition of an emotion in the light of experience, and its impact on the meanings of other concepts such as wrongdoing. This is exactly what we find in the work of Greenspan who analyzes guilt in relation to dilemmas in great depth.[39]

Greenspan believes guilt provides strong evidence that some persons have faced dilemmas. In her view, the guilt faced by persons trapped in dilemmas is not like survivor's guilt, because such persons feel guilty for what they have done. Greenspan also exonerates persons in dilemmas by saying that they are guilty but not blameworthy. On her view, guilt is self-imposed whereas third parties levy blame.[40] Presumably, Sophie and other persons caught in dilemmas may appropriately experience guilt, but third parties do not have the right to blame them.

According to Greenspan, many people are resistant to accepting the reality of dilemmas because they do not want to blame persons trapped in dilemmas. Greenspan believes that many of us falsely assume that correct appraisals of wrongdoing imply that a person acted in a way that was morally worse than another available option. Once we reject this assumption, the evidence based on our emotional lives compels us to accept the reality of dilemmas.[41]

Greenspan offers a sophisticated defense of dilemmas. She has a way of exonerating persons trapped in dilemmas, but her account is acceptable only if her view of first party and third party assessments of persons facing dilemmas makes sense. If we are willing to exonerate other persons in dilemmas, why should it be rational for us to experience guilt for failing to satisfy all moral requirements when we cannot do so? Conversely, if we can be guilty for whatever we do in a dilemma, why would we exonerate another person similarly situated? By exonerating persons in dilemmas, Greenspan has not offered us a position that is substantively different from some dilemma opponents.

Dilemma defenders are fond of adducing moral phenomenology, especially our emotional lives, as evidence for dilemmas. My personal reflections suggest otherwise. All other things remaining equal, I feel different when I intentionally do something wrong; when I intentionally omit to do something I ought to do; when I neglect to do something I ought to do; and when I am incapable of doing something that I would do if I had the ability. True, I must be careful about extrapolating from my experiences to those who face difficult decisions with life and death consequences. Given the vast array of moral circumstances, I am not even sure that my reactions and judgments of my actions and omissions would be consistent. I believe that we should pause before accepting the conclusion that persons in difficult and conflicting circumstances ought to feel guilty and that they face dilemmas. It would help to hear the words of persons trapped in putative dilemmas, but we must interpret and evaluate their remarks among several considerations.

It makes sense that Sinnott-Armstrong believes semantic differences underlie the dispute over the existence of dilemmas. This appears true for those engaged in the accomodationist project. I will next address Sinnott-Armstrong's belief that some situations are dilemmas due to residual requirements to alleviate the losses from our choices.

9. Residual Requirements to Act

Many philosophers divide moral actions into required actions, merely permissible actions, and supererogatory actions in which persons go beyond what is required. Prior to the dilemma debate, conventional wisdom dictated that when a person fails to act upon a moral requirement, the person has done wrong. Possible actions that are permissible but not required carry no moral censure when not carried out. Supererogatory actions are not required and do not warrant blame if not performed. Conversely, supererogatory actions warrant praise when performed. These distinctions between permissible, obligatory, and supererogatory actions and their implications are crude but they allow us to understand Sinnott-Armstrong's position that a person might knowingly transgress a moral requirement without doing wrong.[42] This is a main point in his defense of the existence of dilemmas.

It sounds strange to say that one may transgress a moral requirement without doing wrong, but Sinnott-Armstrong's account is consistent once we understand his distinctions among types of requirements: overriding, overridden, and non-overridden. For him, the only requirements that justify evaluations of wrongdoing when transgressed are overriding requirements. An overriding requirement prescribes an action that ranks morally higher than any other action that is either required or merely permissible. The overriding requirement is what a person ought to perform all things considered.

By contrast, an overridden requirement ranks less high and a person should not perform it. This may be a bit confusing, so let me take a moment to clarify the point.

Sinnott-Armstrong thinks conflicting non-overridden requirements constitute dilemmas.[43] Moral reasons can generate non-overridden requirements strong enough to make moral demands by prescribing an action, but do not rank morally higher than all other possible actions. An alternative can rank higher than a requirement, even an overriding requirement because a supererogatory action may rank higher, but it does not make a moral demand on us in the sense of warranting disapproval if not performed. Again, supererogatory actions go beyond what is required; they are the stuff of special gestures and sainthood. Although Sinnott-Armstrong does not believe the failure to act on a non-overridden requirement entails wrongdoing, he does defend calling the alternatives in dilemmas "requirements" in some strong sense because the failure to satisfy a requirement leads to residual requirements.

To illustrate the concept of a residual requirement, Sinnott-Armstrong has us imagine a bomber pilot who contemplates the possibility of bombing a village hiding enemy soldiers.[44] If the pilot bombs the village, Sinnott-Armstrong says the pilot has a special moral requirement to help the surviving villagers, if any, after the bombing, and that such a requirement makes sense only if we say he violated a moral requirement when he bombed them. The requirement to help the victims of the bombing constitutes a residual requirement. His example has obvious shortcomings, but his point is understandable.

The existence of residual requirements fails to convincingly establish the existence of dilemmas. There appear to be circumstances where one requirement overrides a conflicting alternative that yields a requirement to repair or compensate for the moral loss resulting from the neglected option. Suppose, for instance, that the troops he defended were crucial to preventing the spread of terrorism. On the assumption that the war is justifiable and that overtaking the village is crucial to attaining the ends of just war, the pilot may have an overriding requirement to bomb the village. Still, the pilot may have a special requirement to help the devastated villagers if the opportunity arises. Dilemmas do not appear necessary to explain residual requirements, if we take dilemmas to consist of conflicting non-overridden requirements. After all, in this case, bombing the village is the overriding choice. A glaring challenge with this response to Sinnott-Armstrong's account remains; how does a requirement develop from omitting to perform an overridden act?

Two of the best attempts to account for residual requirements without positing dilemmas belong to Donagan and McConnell. Donagan claims dilemma defenders fail to understand the nature of moral rules, the codification of some requirements. According to Donagan, we should realize that situations can nullify or cancel moral rules.[45]

Donagan believes that persons can place themselves in situations where wrongdoing is inevitable through previous wrongdoing. He leaves us wondering how canceled rules expressing requirements can provide the basis for residue. His answer is that when we face conflicting evaluations of actions due to our wrongdoing, just because we perform one act does not cancel the other option.[46] The problem with Donagan's position, as McConnell notes, is that accounting for residue when circumstances annul or cancel a requirement remains puzzling. What about instances of residue that result from situations where an individual was not guilty of previous wrongdoing? McConnell offers another approach.

McConnell has us imagine a situation wherein we must choose between keeping a trivial promise to meet friends for a routine dinner engagement and saving a person's life.[47] Let us add to his example by saying that a transplant surgeon gets a call that a suitable organ has come available for a patient. To fulfill requirements of professional responsibility, the surgeon is morally required to save the patient's life.

According to McConnell, morality does not require the surgeon to offer compensation or make amends for failing to make the dinner engagement.[48] Instead, the surgeon owes an explanation for not attending, and offering the explanation in no way suggests the surgeon violated a moral requirement.[49] McConnell provides two good reasons for thinking the person did not violate a requirement, and was not in a dilemma. First, the person is not guilty of wrongdoing. Second, saving the person is the unique morally correct response to the situation. In this way, McConnell attempts to explain the presence of a residual requirement, the surgeon's requirement to explain being absent from the dinner engagement without positing dilemmas. McConnell's reasons are plausible, but he also has a problem of explaining residual requirements from cases that do not involve dilemmas.

Even if we agree with McConnell that this example does not constitute a dilemma, it still leaves us wondering how non-dilemmatic cases lead to residual requirements. That is the core challenge to dilemma opponents. Can we explain how a residual requirement develops from a situation where a person does not violate a requirement? Why should we refer to such requirements as residual requirements? Contra McConnell, why not say that even overridden moral reasons generate residue and that we should call such circumstances dilemmas? If this again sounds like a semantic quibble, why does McConnell so adamantly argue against the existence of dilemmas? What we need is a broader explanatory framework as to how requirements develop in cases of moral conflict and cases without moral conflict, but I will not undertake this effort is this book. The issue is complex and raises questions about the extent of the conceptual adequacy of residue.

10. Can We Do Without Residue?

Both defenders and opponents of dilemmas face difficulties when trying to account for all forms of residue—negative emotions and residual requirements and absolve persons who perform well in conflicts. Dilemma defenders have difficulty with absolving agents; opponents with explaining the development of residual requirements. With these difficulties, we may be inclined to call into question the adequacy of the concept of residue. Interestingly, I know of no one who questions or challenges the conceptual adequacy of residue regardless of his or her position on the existence of dilemmas. We have to wonder why parties to the dilemma debate act as if residue is an agreed upon moral datum or set of data for which they need to account.

At one level, both defenders and opponents of dilemmas appear to mean the same thing by residue since all parties to the dilemma debate believe in residue-producing conflicts. Commentators may provisionally agree on the meanings of terms to initiate discussion without meaning the same things by those same terms once they debate the implications of the concepts. When considering cases such as whether persons feel guilt or mere regret over decisions made in tough conflicts or whether a person such as the surgeon who misses the dinner party to save another's life has a requirement to make amends or merely to offer an explanation for being absent, disagreements over the implications of residue are relevant. Participants to the debate agree about the presence of some sort of residue, but disagree as to whether it implies a dilemma or a conflict.

Though residue may not beg the question in favor of dilemmas, "residual requirement" hardly sounds theoretically neutral. But how can we not refer to the results of some conflicts as residual requirements when we have strong reasons to make amends of some sort, to feel badly about what has happened, or to avoid similar circumstances in the future? Can we embrace the concept of residue without implying the existence of residual requirements? If we reject the concept of residue, how should we describe the negative moral consequences of conflicting values? Have we taken the metaphor of residue too seriously? Is all this talk about residue merely a dramatic, misleading way of saying that some of our requirements result from previous acts?

Our current requirements linking past circumstances and commitments with current affairs and future goals are not surprising or controversial. Both defenders and opponents of dilemmas need to acknowledge the flow of the moral life, but we should consider whether the concept of residue proves to be more problematic than helpful.

Consider a physician who must decide which of two patients to save. Even if the doctor makes a justified decision to save one patient, there will be reasons and a requirement to save the other patient too, if the opportunity arises. If the other patient dies, the doctor may owe an explanation and an apology to the dead patient's family. Instead of saying a dilemmatic situation generated a residual requirement for the physician to provide an explanation and to apologize, we can say that the new condition of the world creates the requirement—the patient's death and the presence of the patient's family. Under this description, there would be no explicit appeal to residue. But how do we know whether we are implicitly appealing to residue?

One problem with the attempt to explain away the existence of a residual requirement is that it may prove too much. It also suggests the non-existence of a residual reason to mollify the harm of an action. If the new condition of the world forms the basis of new requirements, then after we perform an action, the new condition of the world also forms the basis of moral reasons such as recommendations. If residual reasons to perform an act or to adopt an attitude do not exist, there can be no type of residue-producing conflict.

We know, however, that values conflict and that these conflicts produce moral losses and that these losses provide us with reasons to make the world a better place. If we admit residual reasons, I see no plausible reason for denying the existence of residual requirements. For these reasons, I think we implicitly appeal to residue so long as we acknowledge the continuity of moral requirements and reasons that stem from losses that result from previous choices. I provisionally accept the notion of residue even though the dilemma debate and the accommodationist project have not been resolved to my satisfaction.

11. Conclusion

The preceding debate over the possibility of facing incompatible requirements leaves us with several interesting but difficult puzzles. Embracing dilemmas suggests that a person can be wrong and blameworthy even when the person does the best that circumstances allow. Rejecting dilemmas leaves us with difficulties explaining the concept of a residual requirement. Without a heroic effort to dispense with the concept of residue, we need the concept of residue to understand significant features of our moral lives. Whatever our opinion on the existence of dilemmas, I recommend that we take a practical approach by acknowledging that residue-producing conflicts exist and that these conflicts leave us with requirements and reasons to make amends, to explain ourselves, to avoid future conflicts, and to experience emotions such as regret or remorse. As we will see, we will need to make institutional, scientific, technological, psychological, legal, and conceptual adjustments in response to conflicts involving organ retrieval. In turn, responding to these conflicts begets moral losses, residue, and more conflicts.

In the next chapter, I discuss how we might approach conflicts regarding organ retrieval by utilizing the concepts of medical ethics that are widely accepted throughout the world, especially the United States. I discuss the real-life case of Cliff's choice that helps us understand the benefits and limitations of moral concepts. This case is more open ended than the hypothetical cases in the philosophical literature used to illustrate points about dilemmas, conflicts, and residue. Cliff's choice illustrates the identification of values and conflicts, the role of luck and hope, issues about comparing values, and the need for constant interventions in constructing a good life.

Two

MEDICAL ETHICS AND ITS LIMITATIONS

1. Cliff's Choice

Films for the Humanities & Sciences produced a series of videos meant to stimulate our thinking about medical ethics. In the video, "The Decision: Whose Kidney Is It Anyway?" we learn that Cliff Pendregaust has two adult sons, Neil and Russell, who suffer from Alport's syndrome, a disease that has destroyed their kidneys.[1] Neil does not respond well to dialysis. Although Russell responds to dialysis well enough to work as a general manager for a chain of luxury hotels, his treatments absorb fifteen hours per week and diminish his quality of life. Cliff proves to be a compatible donor for both of his sons, but the transplant team rules out his wife, Eva, on medical grounds. Cliff faces the choice of donating one of his kidneys to either Neil or Russell.

Cliff's choice provides an interesting parallel to Sophie's choice, but we must note significant disanalogies. As Cliff deliberates on which son should receive his kidney, both his children are adults. Cliff has good reason to believe that in time, both of his sons can find medical help. The outcome of Cliff's choice appears more open-ended than was Sophie's choice. The decision is not Cliff's choice alone, but one made by his entire family. Though Cliff has to decide which of his sons he will help first, Russell makes the decision easier when he admirably recommends that Neil receive the kidney since Neil is in poorer health.

Fortunately, both Neil and Cliff fare well after the surgery. All appears well with Russell too, for he later receives a cadaver kidney. Unfortunately, Russell's transplant fails because an artery connecting his donor kidney to his blood supply bursts. Thereafter, Russell's health slowly deteriorates on dialysis. He needs another transplant, but his previous failed transplant causes him to produce antibodies that make him incompatible with 96% of the population.

In a surprising twist, Cliff offers his remaining kidney to Russell. Cliff reasons that he is old anyway and that dialysis would not appreciably diminish his quality of life. Russell says his father is overreacting, but the entire family apparently agrees to the proposal. Three hospitals refuse to do the surgery. Sue Woods, the transplant coordinator at Middlesex Hospital in London, claims Cliff's sacrifice is too great to justify the surgery. Cliff's quality of life and life expectancy apparently took priority over Cliff's preference to make this sacrifice and the benefit Russell would receive. Consequently, the hospital reconsiders the suitability of Eva as a donor. This time they determine she would make a compatible donor but that her health might not be good enough to justify her being a donor. The video ends without viewers knowing whether Russell will live or die from his illness.

In his book on the legal and ethical issues of organ transplantation David Price noted that in the end Eva donated a kidney to Russell.[2] The makers of the video appear content with raising the ethical issue of whether the transplant team at Middlesex Hospital should have acceded to Cliff's request to give his only kidney to Russell. In what follows, I discuss five notable approaches to medical ethics and the common assumptions of these models. I then return to the case of Cliff's choice.

I will discuss five approaches to medical ethics: the four-principle model of Tom Beauchamp and James Childress, the virtue ethics of Edmund Pellegrino and David Thomasma, feminist ethics, a case-based model of clinical ethics, and Hugo Tristram Engelhardt's postmodern libertarianism. Again, because Beauchamp and Childress present the most popular way of thinking about medical ethics, I will pay special attention to their model.

2. Beauchamp and Childress's Principlism

Beauchamp and Childress offer four ethical principles to follow when considering medical ethical cases or policy questions: respect for patient autonomy, beneficence, nonmaleficence, and justice.[3] In contrast to Beauchamp and Childress, I prefer to discuss medical ethics in terms of values instead of principles, but this difference will not create any problems in explaining their account. Beauchamp and Childress acknowledge that others might develop their principles as rights, virtues, or values in another framework.

Ethical principles are explicit articulations of values meant to guide our moral responses. As such, respect for autonomy calls us to honor the preferences of patients. The value of beneficence indicates that we should promote patients' well-being while nonmaleficence calls us to refrain from harming patients. Justice pertains to giving people what they deserve including fair access to healthcare.

Like William David Ross, Beauchamp and Childress believe that those responsible for people's healthcare have a *prima facie* requirement to fulfill each principle and an actual requirement to fulfill each principle unless the principles conflict. In times of conflict, the point is to determine our requirements given all of the relevant information. For Beauchamp and Childress, conflicts are typical features of the moral life, and so resolving or dissolving conflicts is crucial to leading moral lives. Beauchamp and Childress provide two primary approaches to resolving conflict: specifying and balancing.

Beauchamp and Childress never adequately clarify the concept of specification but they do provide interesting ideas worth considering. According to Beauchamp and Childress, specification provides more concrete moral advice by making norms determinate in content. Since principles are norms, their comment implies that specification makes principles more determinate, but norms include rules and directives as well. They imply a semantic and logical component to specification that involves the meaning and scope of a norm.

As an example of specification, they invite us to consider the rule "Doctors should put their patients' interests first." They point out that in the United States, patients can sometimes afford the best treatment only if their physicians falsify information on insurance forms. Such situations place physicians in the unenviable position of having to choose between patients' best interests and telling the truth or not misleading the insurers. Beauchamp and Childress explain that attempts to determine what constitutes deception and when deception is morally permissible are examples of "attempts to specify rules against deception."[4] In this case, specification appears to involve a semantic and a moral process by which we determine the meaning of deception and when deception is justifiable. Appropriate specification, then, can circumvent the problem of comparing the value of conflicting courses of action by determining whether a moral principle applies in a case.

Specification also provides a way to resolve conflicts. Beauchamp and Childress add, "When moral conflicts occur, specification supplies an ideal of repeated coherence testing and modification of a principle or rule until the conflict is specified away."[5] They clarify that specification cannot eliminate all moral conflict. And, "the method is suited only for contexts in which specification has a reasonable hope of acceptance."[6] They admonish, "making norms specific does not itself preclude the use of dogmatic, biased, arbitrary, or irrational views to make one's favored conclusion correct by fiat."[7]

In saying that biases can make a conclusion true by fiat, they mean that we can define moral concepts in a way that leads to desirable conclusions but only at the expense of circular reasoning. What they mean by saying that the method is suited only for contexts where the specification has hope of acceptance is vague. They could mean that the method itself is inappropriate in contexts where acceptance is unlikely or that specification is not appropriate in contexts where a conclusion yielded by the method of specification is unlikely to be accepted. It also remains ambiguous whether specification for such situations is inappropriate based on prudential or moral grounds. Whatever the case, in conjunction with the implied semantic component of specification, so long as specification involves determining whether an action is justifiable, we will be faced with the familiar issue of justifying our moral priorities. For these reasons Beauchamp and Childress say, "Nothing in the model of specification indicates a way around balancing in the very act of specifying principles and rules."[8]

Whereas specification involves the meaning and scope of norms, Beauchamp and Childress claim that balancing justifies moral judgments. In their words, "balancing consists of deliberation and judgment about the relative weights of norms."[9] An individual's obligation is determined by balancing the respective weights of competing *prima facie* obligations. The heavier of the competing obligations is the one that takes priority, the overriding obligation upon which a person should act.

Beauchamp and Childress insist that the weighing metaphor should not mislead us into thinking that balancing is intuitive or subjective. They say, justified balancing entails that we provide good reasons for our judgments. In this way, the problem of different individuals having different intuitions will not lead to a moral stalemate. Though what constitutes a good reason is not evident, they do provide ways to overcome intuitive and subjective judgments when balancing conflicting values. To overcome the problem that balancing is too "intuitive and open-ended," they offer five conditions to justify overriding one *prima facie* norm in favor of another *prima facie* norm.

First, the reasons for infringing upon a norm must be better than the reasons for upholding that norm. For instance, the value of protecting a person's right to something is more heavily weighted against persons who have an interest in that same thing but do not have a right to that thing. A person might have an interest in another person's kidney, but the person does not have a right to another person's kidney. Second, the objective justifying the infringement of a *prima facie* norm must have a realistic prospect of achievement. Doctors can only respect the prohibition against harming patients in the case of living kidney transplants if saving the lives of both the donor and the recipient can be successful. Third, there can be no preferable alternative action for an action that constitutes a violation of a norm. If a physician has an obligation to care for a patient, and transplantation would benefit the patient more than dialysis, then all other things remaining equal, transplantation would be the appropriate course. Fourth, the extent of the infringement is the least possible. Fifth, minimize the negative effects of the infringement.

Beauchamp and Childress need to distinguish between minimizing infringements and making sure that an infringement is the least possible, but we can understand the moral appropriateness of minimizing the ill effects of moral losses created by our choices—that is the exact point of moral residue. They believe that these minimal conditions help in protecting against "arbitrary, purely intuitive judgments" even though determining which norm deserves priority will not always be possible. They insist that balancing is justifiable only upon the presentation of adequate reasons.

These remarks give us a lot to consider. I will not respond to each of their five conditions for balancing conflicting principles, but addressing their efforts to minimize intuitive judgments is crucial. True, we should attempt to provide reasons for our beliefs. A problem with their account is that the criteria they utilize to limit intuitive judgments are vague or debatable when applied to a real-life case. Consider their use of phrases such as "realistic prospect for achievement," "no morally preferable action," and "adequate reasons" to help us decide which courses of action are morally required or morally permissible. What is supposed to count as a realistic prospect for achievement regarding the xenotransplantation of whole organs or stem cell research? It cannot be that such efforts can presently help many patients with failing organs, and if that were the criterion, virtually no novel therapy could be justified. On the other hand, if adding to the corpus of medical knowledge constitutes an achievement, no matter how modest, virtually every therapy could be justified.

What judgments can avoid these two extremes? Depending on the context, such as clinical trials or experimental treatments, we will need to develop rules that are more precise—what Beauchamp and Childress would rightfully want. The persistence of moral debate indicates that the lack of more precise rules or reasons is not the only difficulty in resolving debate or justifying a course of action. Many rules and reasons remain debatable or vacuous. For example, we know not to subject persons to unnecessary medical risks, but how does this principle apply in the case of Cliff Pendregaust? In many cases, what constitutes a morally preferable alternative is elusive. We must also wonder how frequently Beauchamp and Childress believe circumstances allow for the determination of an overriding norm so that we can show one action among many to be required or morally best. Without a model for determining overriding norms in most cases, competing intuitions will be inevitable.

Although Beauchamp and Childress say that we will not find a perfect belief system, they probably believe that we can usually determine overriding norms for specified circumstances. Most of their moral skepticism targets moral theory, not moral decisions, even though their skepticism regarding moral theory has ramifications for decision-making. In their words, "it is unreasonable to expect any theory to overcome all the limitations of time and place and reach a universally acceptable perspective."[10] Consistent with this skepticism, they say, "ethics of public policy must proceed from impure and unsettled cases, in which there are profound social disagreements, uncertainties, different interpretations of history, and imperfect procedures to resolve the disagreements."[11] They do not elaborate on these imperfect procedures or even identify the procedures to which they refer. Based upon their other comments, they apparently mean procedures involving the correct application of the aforementioned principles to a case or policy.

Beauchamp and Childress expect people to disagree sometimes about an issue even after thorough analysis. They claim that moral principles can conflict and produce dilemmas that may resist resolution even after careful consideration. They say, "abstract rules and principles in moral theories are extensively indeterminate."[12] By "indeterminate," they apparently mean that decision makers cannot find or develop a solution, presumably a single best solution, to a problem. To overcome this indeterminacy, they say we must consider the facts, cultural expectations, judgments of likely outcome, and precedents previously encountered:

even if we have our facts straight, the choice of facts and the choice of rules will generate a judgment that is incompatible with another choice of facts and rules. Obtaining the right set of facts and bringing the right set of rules to bear on these facts are not reducible either to a deductive form of judgment or to the resources of a general ethical theory.[13]

Paying attention to circumstances allows us to overcome the indeterminateness of theory but not entirely.

Contra the views of many commentators on dilemmas and conflicts, Beauchamp and Childress leave us with the impression that these difficulties stem from the limitations of theory, not of conflicting impositions of the world. They buttress this suspicion by saying, "To the surprise of many philosophers in the last twenty years, often little is lost in practical moral decision-making by dispensing with general moral theories."[14] The reason for their view is, "the rules and principles shared across these theories typically serve practical judgment more adequately . . . than the theories."[15] At the same time, they recognize that principles are general guides that leave considerable room for judgment regarding cases.

How should we interpret "considerable room for judgment" if not as the view that principles will also yield indeterminate answers in circumstances, thereby leaving individual decision-makers to their knowledge, experience, intuitions, and prejudices? What are we to do about the selection of different facts and rules? How do we choose well or know which theories, principles, and judgments are true?

Fortunately, Beauchamp and Childress clarify their preferred epistemological framework for addressing these questions. They accept the epistemological model of reflective equilibrium whereby both our principles and our judgments are subject to revision or outright rejection in the light of further reflection and evidence.[16] In their words:

> we start with paradigm judgments of moral rightness and wrongness, and then construct a more general theory that is consistent with these paradigm judgments (so that they are as coherent as possible); any loopholes are closed, as are all forms of incoherence that are detected. The resultant action-guides are then tested to see if they too yield incoherent results. If so, they are readjusted or given up, and the process is renewed, because we can never assume a completely stable equilibrium.[17]

When principles lead to counter-intuitive conclusions, or our intuitions appear awry, we should make revisions until theories, principles, and judgments are consistent. Although Beauchamp and Childress do not say so, a coherent set of beliefs consists of logical and explanatory connections between beliefs.

Otherwise, we could have a coherent set of statements that are unrelated. With that emendation in mind, Beauchamp and Childress believe, "all moral systems present some level of indeterminateness and incoherence, revealing that they do not have the power to eliminate different contingent conflicts among principles and rules."[18] For this reason, "there is no reason to anticipate that the process of pruning, adjusting, and rendering coherent will either come to an end or be perfected."[19]

We should not expect perfection in terms of always being able to find determinate answers to questions about ethical theory or ethical judgments or discovering answers that always will be consistent. Instead, we should understand, "Every general norm, indeed morality itself, contains regions of indeterminacy that need reduction through further development and enrichment."[20] What we have is an, "evolving moral life."[21] Even though Beauchamp and Childress point out some of our limitations with moral decision-making, they do not emphasize the point when discussing cases and policies.

In summary, we can understand their model as consisting of the following key features. First, they are pluralists in the sense that they offer four principles to guide us with our decision-making regarding medical ethics: autonomy, beneficence, nonmaleficence, and justice. Second, we should act upon each of these four principles when relevant, unless one principle overrides a conflicting principle. Third, to determine whether one principle overrides another principle, we must subject the principles to a process of specification and balancing. The principle with the most weight overrides the other principle with which it conflicts and is the principle upon which we should act. Fourth, to prevent the weighing process from being too intuitive, we must develop and apply precise rules to cases. That, in a nutshell, is the Beauchamp and Childress model of medical ethics, the model that dominates American medical ethics.

Pellegrino and Thomasma help explain why the Beauchamp and Childress model has been so influential. They write:

> The four-principle approach has been taught to thousands of health professionals through the most popular intensive bioethics course, conducted annually by the faculty of the Kennedy Institute of Ethics for the last seventeen years. Through its 200 or so graduates per year, this course has had a strong influence on the teaching and research of health professionals and ethicists who teach in medical schools, colleges and universities, or consult in clinical settings. Many younger health professionals have learned ethics from those graduates, who now head up many of the centers of bioethics. The four-principle tradition is now so widely accepted that some of its more whimsical critics have labeled it a "mantra," applied automatically and without sound moral grounding.[22]

In 1993, Pellegrino and Thomasma claimed that there has been a backlash against Beauchamp and Childress's principlism. But ten years later, their model remains the dominant one in the United States, especially, the ethics work of healthcare providers.[23]

Others offer alternative approaches to medical ethics, but many of these authors share significant views with Beauchamp and Childress. Pellegrino and Thomasma offer a medical ethics model based on virtue ethics, and speak of the importance of justice, autonomy, and beneficence. Feminist ethicists emphasize maintaining relationships and the abuse of power, but accept many of the same moral concepts as Beauchamp and Childress. Others offer a model of casuistry that develops moral principles based on judgments made about cases.

Even those who believe that they offer a different approach to medical ethics are heavily reliant on Beauchamp and Childress. We see this, for example, in the work of Albert Jonsen, Mark Siegler, and William J. Winslade who emphasize the importance of detail to cases.[24] H. Tristram Engelhardt addresses the limits of Beauchamp and Childress's model, but he offers a two-principle system of autonomy and beneficence. All of these medical ethicists discuss the conflict of different principles and the difficulties with weighing and balancing principles. Although many have challenged the Beauchamp and Childress model, the core remains intact.

3. Virtue Ethics

Although Pellegrino and Thomasma appreciate Beauchamp and Childress's four-principle model, they encourage us to supplement the model because the way principles are interpreted, ranked, and applied depends on an individual's character.[25] People need to develop virtuous character, for good principles are neither necessary nor sufficient for ethical conduct. They advise:

> one may have a good grasp of ethical principles and yet not apply them correctly or in a dependable way; on the other hand, there are persons of character who may not be aware of moral principles or may even reason incorrectly about them, but are of such character that they can be depended upon to act rightly.[26]

According to Pellegrino and Thomasma, Beauchamp and Childress's four principles stem from obligations owed by physicians to their patients. By contrast, they offer a medical ethics model centered on the patient-physician relationship where physicians are encouraged to exemplify the virtues of compassion, justice, fortitude, temperance, integrity, self-effacement, and prudence. Of these virtues, prudence receives special attention for the way it guides persons to correct behavior in the light of all virtues. Pellegrino and Thomasma especially encourage physicians to develop virtuous character, for physicians possess medical authority and patients are needy and vulnerable. In the United States, all healthcare providers should cultivate virtuous character because patients often spend more time with nurses, physician assistants, and medical aides than with physicians.

Pellegrino and Thomasma suggest that the Beauchamp and Childress model fails for other reasons as well. For one, they believe that the four principles lack theoretical grounding in a great tradition of moral philosophy such as utilitarianism, deontology, virtue ethics, or even better, the clinical encounter. I prefer plausible free-floating principles to implausible moral traditions. Besides, someone could make a serious attempt to ground the principles in a great tradition, but I will not undertake this effort.

Second, and more to the point of this book, Pellegrino and Thomasma believe that Beauchamp and Childress overemphasize the conflict of principles. They say, for example, that respecting the autonomy of the patient does not conflict with beneficence toward the patient, because acting contrary to the patient's autonomy is maleficent. They apparently have in mind cases where a patient refuses medical treatment that would be helpful. They do not have a case like Cliff's choice in mind where things are more complicated. In that example, we must consider ethical conduct related to two patients. Failing to act in accordance with Cliff's and Russell's choice to undergo a kidney transplant may lead to Russell's harm or death. Refusing to act in accordance with their autonomy is for beneficent reasons.

Third, they believe that the model of balancing *prima facie* principles might oversimplify decisions. Other times, *prima facie* principles provide too little guidance. Their criticism of *prima facie* principles is more interesting for my purposes and deserves greater attention.

Pellegrino and Thomasma correctly identify the problem with adjudicating among conflicting *prima facie* principles. They wonder whether the justification of overriding a principle rests on another *prima facie* principle or the circumstances of an ethical choice. In either case, they believe that relying on *prima facie* principles is problematic. "If it is another prima facie principle, then we face the problem of one principle having greater moral weight than another. There is no formal mechanism or convincing argument that would grant trumping privileges to one principle over another."[27] If the circumstances justify an ethical choice, "the circumstances themselves would take on the moral force of a *prima facie* principle, or they would have to be justified by one of the *prima facie* principles—but which one?"[28] They note that the Beauchamp and Childress's model pits the *prima facie* principles against one another. According to Pellegrino and Thomasma, attempting to resolve a conflict between *prima facie* principles leads to circular reasoning.

Unfortunately, Pellegrino and Thomasma fail to explain why balancing *prima facie* principles inevitably leads to fallacious reasoning. As we will see with the discussion of the weighing metaphor in the next chapter, some of our moral judgments can be justified without appeal to formal mechanisms or any great mysteries about the relationship between the weight of a *prima facie* principle and circumstances. Pellegrino and Thomasma have identified a significant problem with ethics in general and Beauchamp and Childress's model especially, how do we weigh our options?

Despite the substantial problem with weighing conflicting *prima facie* principles or values, Pellegrino and Thomasma choose to accommodate instead of abandon the Beauchamp and Childress four-principle model. They accommodate the principles of autonomy, beneficence, and justice because even virtuous individuals will need principles to guide behavior. Pellegrino and Thomasma eloquently defend the principle of autonomy. In their words:

> Autonomy has particular appeal in medical relationships. It counters the historical dominance of benign authoritarianism or paternalism in the traditional ethics of medicine. It ensures that patients may choose among treatment alternatives, accept or reject any of them, and thus retain control over some of the most intimate and personal decisions in their lives. Respect for autonomy also protects patients against submergence of their moral values and beliefs. In morally diverse societies where physicians and patients may have markedly different cultural, ethnic, and religious origins, observance of this facet of autonomy is especially and justifiably cherished.[29]

Although Pellegrino and Thomasma attempt to argue that conflicts between autonomy and beneficence are more apparent than real, they recognize conflicts between autonomy and justice. Such conflicts extend to the virtues as well. They remind us, "at every junction, some prudential assessment of competing values, principles, or virtues must be made."[30] On another occasion they claim, "It is often a painful task to constantly adjust and balance conflicting needs and goods . . . at every junction, some prudential assessment of competing values, principles, or virtues must be made."[31]

In response to the conflicts between principles, values, and virtues, Pellegrino and Thomasma believe we pay too little attention to good clinical judgment that comes through the cultivation of the virtue of prudence. Since formal mechanisms cannot determine precisely what a physician should do when confronted with a moral conflict, prudence enables, "the physician to assess the relative weight of the means at her disposal, the therapeutic possibilities, and outcomes and side effects, and the values and life circumstances of the patient, as well as his preferences and other factors."[32]

In the final analysis, virtue theory does complement the Beauchamp and Childress model for the reasons claimed by Pellegrino and Thomasma. Without virtue, persons may lack the motivation to act in accordance with principles. Even though Pellegrino and Thomasma tell us that the Beauchamp and

Childress model is under attack and even though they anticipate the future erosion of its influence, still, they reinforce much of the heart of the Beauchamp and Childress model. As has been shown, they accept the principles of autonomy, beneficence, and justice; they acknowledge the conflict of principles, values, and virtues; and they recognize the need to weigh and balance conflicting principles, values, and virtues. This is a recurring theme in criticisms of Beauchamp and Childress: commentators supplement instead of reject their model. Even when medical ethicists reject much of Beauchamp and Childress's perspective, they retain significant premises.

4. Feminist Bioethics

Carol Gilligan's influential book, *In a Different Voice: Psychological Theory and Women's Development*, paved the way for feminist ethics and its application to many contemporary moral problems.[33] According to Gilligan, interviews with males and females of different ages show that males tend to think of morality in terms of justice whereby persons need to adjudicate conflicting principles. Females tend to think in terms of care in which they seek ways to maintain relationships and account for all persons' needs. Feminist bioethics incorporates the elements of care ethics and analyzes moral issues in terms of the power relations of those involved. In this section, I summarize the thoughts of two prominent feminist bioethicists, Rosemarie Tong and Susan Sherwin, who consider the subordination of women in healthcare systems, and the way we interpret and address problems within medical ethics.

Tong recognizes several feminist perspectives, but identifies two forms of feminist ethics, care-based ethics and power-based ethics.[34] Care-based ethics or care ethics emphasizes traditional virtues associated with women and femininity such as care and compassion. Power-based ethics addresses the institutions and systems that continue to subjugate women. Within care ethics and power-based ethics, Tong identifies four themes emerging from feminist scholarship: eclecticism in politics, autokoenomy in ontology, positionality in epistemology, and relationality in ethics. Political eclecticism allows feminists the wherewithal to draw from many political traditions such as liberalism, socialism, Marxism, and radical feminism. Autokoenomy emphasizes that individual selves are part of a network of relationships, so an individual must make choices with several people in mind. Regarding epistemology, Tong describes positionalists as those who believe that although "there is truth to be known, knowledge of this truth is always situational and partial."[35] Relational ethics emphasizes the desire to maintain good, freely chosen relationships, and the need to overcome coercive relationships. How do these themes help us think about medical ethics?

Sherwin claims that most feminists reject the abstract-principle model in favor of a contextual model. She notes that traditional ethical theories such as utilitarianism and deontology consider the context of ethical decision-making to determine whether a principle applies in a case and how to fulfill a principle. Feminist contextualism focuses on applying and fulfilling principles by close attention to details, considering the relationships between the relevant parties, and the political and historical context of decisions. Sherwin believes we should strive to eliminate all forms of oppression, but medical ethics has not made a commitment to ending oppression. According to Sherwin, mainstream medical ethics is complicitous with oppression. In her words:

> Most debates in bioethics have focused on specific matters of concern within the existing healthcare system, such as truthfulness, consent, confidentiality, the limits of paternalism, the allocation of resources, incurable illness, and abortion. The effect of this narrow orientation has been to provide an overall ethical legitimization of the existing healthcare institutions, whereas general structures and patterns are left largely unchallenged.[36]

But how do feminist insights impact our view of organ retrieval strategies? According to Sherwin, a feminist analysis of medical practices must include medical views of the human body. In words that are provocative for the transplant community she says:

> Patients are required to submit to medical authority and respond with gratitude for attention offered. Most recognize their vulnerability to medical power and learn the value of offering a cheerful disposition in the face of extraordinary suffering, because complaints are often met with hostility and impatience . . . . Medical practice involves the explorative study, manipulation, and modification of the body; because, under patriarchal ideology, the body is characteristically associated with the feminine, the female body is particularly subject to medical dominance.[37]

At the same time, organ transplantation manifests an extraordinary effort to heal the human body. Precisely how feminist ethics should influence our view of organ transplantation is indefinite.

Sherwin also emphasizes that "medicine should be transformed from one principally occupied with crisis management to one primarily committed to fostering health empowerment."[38] Given the incredibly invasive nature of organ retrieval and transplantation and post-transplant suffering, we must wonder when the scientific and medical community will develop better approaches to treating organ failure. I will revisit the suggestion to improve preventive medicine strategies in chapter ten.

Feminist bioethics as advanced by Tong and Sherwin are genuine, significant contributions to the field of medical ethics and has the greatest potential for changing medical ethics and the healthcare system for the better. But we need to note differences between the work of Tong and Sherwin and my work. First, neither Tong nor Sherwin emphasizes the problem with the incommensurability of values that is central to my work. As I will show, part of the difficulty with comparing the value of alternative courses of action is that the good action is not always to be found by careful reflection and dialogue but is to be made through on-going ventures. I accept the importance of relational ethics and the fallibilism of positionalist epistemology. Some answers are not there to discover. Ethics involves the attempt to realize potential future states of affairs through a series of intelligent efforts.

Despite its potential for radical reform, feminist medical ethics shares insights with the Beauchamp and Childress model. For example, Sherwin's position does not entail that principles are irrelevant or that Beauchamp and Childress's principles are inapplicable. Sherwin acknowledges that many feminists accept that principles are significant for ethics. She adds, "my argument against oppression is a principled one."[39] She challenges mainstream applications of ethical principles by claiming, "it is assumed, all the relevant features of a particular case can be clarified in a short description of its features."[40] Point taken. She also accepts the weighing metaphor and by saying that claims must be balanced; she assumes that there will be conflicting ethical concerns. She states, for instance, that both medical ethics and feminist ethics assign special weight to ethical concerns such as caring and responsibility. Sherwin adds that care ethics offers norms for balancing obligations related to self and others. Feminists do not always agree as to what policies and practices we should adopt or permit, so we will look to other models to help us make good decisions.

5. Case Analysis

Some medical ethicists propose case analysis as an alternative to the principlism of Beauchamp and Childress. Alluding to Beauchamp and Childress's model, Jonsen, Siegler, and Winslade claim, "Many books on healthcare ethics are organized around moral principles, such as respect for autonomy, beneficence, nonmaleficence, and fairness. The cases are analyzed in the light of those principles. Our method is different."[41] These authors believe that the case-based method better captures the complexities of clinical realities in a straightforward way.

We need to discern how these defenders of case analysis propose that their method is different. They set forth two issues to distinguish their method from that of Beauchamp and Childress and merely allude to other differences. First, they claim that healthcare providers should analyze every case with respect to medical indications, patient preferences, quality of life, and contextual features. Second, they say, "Our method of analysis begins, not with the principles and rules, as do many other ethics treatises, but with the factual features of the case."[42] They suggest that their method is different because other methods discuss principles in an abstract way while their presentation avoids the tendency to "think of only one principle as the sole guide in the case."[43] We can infer that they believe their method is more concrete and more sophisticated in that they recognize the influence of a plurality of relevant principles for application to cases.

It turns out that the method of Jonsen, Siegler, and Winslade is not that different from the method of Beauchamp and Childress. Like Beauchamp and Childress, they mention the relevance of the principles of respect for autonomy, beneficence, nonmaleficence, and justice. In addition, they include a principle of loyalty defined as "a sustained commitment to the welfare of persons or to the success of an endeavor, requiring an investment of effort and sometimes even a subordination of self-interest."[44] They also mention a principle of respect for persons, but they do not clarify how this principle differs from a principle of autonomy. They indicate that the principles of beneficence and nonmaleficence are significant guides to meet the goals of medicine and that respect for patients' preferences honors the principle of autonomy.

Although their language is different, Jonsen, Siegler, and Winslade appear to accept Beauchamp and Childress's claims regarding specification and balancing. For example, they state that the medical realities of a case such as the compromised competence of a patient and the stress of illness can limit the realization of patient autonomy. This point sounds like what Beauchamp and Childress claimed about specification: that the scope of a principle may not apply to a case. Jonsen, Siegler, and Winslade also recognize that one value can take priority over another value, that one value can override the other value. This is what Beauchamp and Childress say about balancing conflicting values. Thinking that their method is different because they begin with the facts of a case instead of with the principles is like thinking you get a different meal depending on whether you eat the dessert or the entrée first.

Jonsen, Siegler, and Winslade also use the weighing metaphor. When discussing whether to disclose unpleasant information to a patient, they say that the value of knowledge outweighs the short-term value of ignorance. When considering whether to honor parents' right to determine the healthcare of their children, they say, "it is sometimes necessary to determine the relevance and weight of parental preferences when these preferences conflict with the recommendations of providers."[45] Jonsen, Siegler, and Winslade have more in common with Beauchamp and Childress than they acknowledge.

Other facets of Jonsen, Siegler, and Winslade's work invite exploration for its suggestions concerning the incommensurability of values and the plurality of right action. When it comes to making good decisions regarding a clinical case, they believe that rational choices must account for patient preferences and medical indications. They say, "there are often several medically reasonable options for treating a particular problem, and each option is associated with different risks and benefits for the patient,"[46] adding, "different patients may express quite different but entirely reasonable preferences when faced with the same medical indications."[47]

Jonsen, Siegler, and Winslade are correct in saying that different patients can make different good choices in similar circumstances. Patients will have good reason to select one option as the best for them depending on what sorts of risks they are willing to take, how much pain and suffering they are willing to endure, or how a treatment regimen will affect their work or family life. At times, the patient's cultural background will dictate the best course of action for that patient. Although they generally advocate disclosing risks to patients, they point out that Navajo Indians believe that language determines reality and so individual Navajos speak positively for fear that negative remarks will cause bad outcomes. They recommend healthcare providers should shield from a Navajo the potential negative effects of a treatment regimen in a case where the risk of harm is slight. Even if readers disagree with this particular example as an exception to the principle of autonomy, the example illustrates how right action varies with context and individual differences.

The emphasis that Jonsen, Siegler, and Winslade give to respect for patients helps explain why many medical ethicists do not frequently discuss the incommensurability of values. It makes sense to believe that patients must value options that they choose over other options. Otherwise, it would be difficult to understand why they made that choice as opposed to alternatives.

Honoring patient preferences shifts the burden of comparing values from healthcare providers and medical ethicists to patients. This is not to say that healthcare providers and medical ethicists will not have an intuitive or well-formed opinion about the best alternative available to a patient. Allowing patients to make decisions that directly affect them is appropriate. We should allow individuals to make decisions that we would judge to be bad decisions. By honoring patient preferences, healthcare providers and medical ethicists escape the burden of trying to prioritize the value of alternative actions.

How do patients know what is best for them, even after they have the needed medical information? At times, they will have a good understanding as to which option they should select, but other times they will not be in any better position to compare the relevant values than would anyone else appraising the situation. Many questions regarding medical ethics and the ethics of organ retrieval involve policy questions that impact local communities, nations, and the international community. For this reason, we need to better understand the reasons, decision procedures, capabilities, and limitations of comparing the moral value of alternative courses of action.

Even when medical ethicists acknowledge situations in which they find good reasons for more than one alternative, the desire to find the best response is strong. Jonsen, Siegler, and Winslade consider a case in which a young man appears to have bacterial meningitis, yet the man adamantly and mysteriously refuses treatment even after he has been told repeatedly of the risk of non-treatment.[48] The question is, should the physicians paternalistically subject the patient to treatment? The authors say:

> The conscientious physician faces two evils: to honor a refusal that might not represent the patient's true preferences, thus leading to the patient's serious disability or death, or to override the refusal in the hope that, subsequently, the patient will recognize the benefit. This is a genuine moral dilemma: The principle of beneficence and the principle of autonomy seem to dictate contradictory courses of action.[49]

They apparently believe that one option is best. As they say, "dilemmas cannot merely be contemplated; they must be resolved . . . we resolve it in favor of treatment against the expressed preferences of this patient."[50] Jonsen, Siegler, and Winslade never clarify what they mean by "resolve," but judging from the context, it means finding a single best solution for a case.

To the credit of Jonsen, Siegler, and Winslade, and in contrast to the vast majority of American articles on medical ethics, they explicitly claim that in some cases more than one option is morally permissible. They consider a case in which a two-day-old infant has a hypoplastic left heart. The infant will die unless a surgical technique called the Norwood procedure successfully repairs the heart or the infant receives a heart transplant. At the time of the publication of their book, 1998, two-thirds of infants who received the Norwood technique survived up to five years after undergoing several surgeries. Conversely, many such infants suffer major disabilities. In this case, the authors believe that parents may justifiably allow the child to die and that they may justifiably consent to the Norwood procedure unless a heart is available for transplantation. They believe either option is permissible even though they believe that the parents should reject the Norwood procedure. Unfortunately, they do not adequately explain why they would reject the Norwood procedure as the best option, while also defending the parents' decision to consent to the Norwood procedure. Significantly, the vast majority of medical ethics discussion assumes a best response for each case or policy question and that our current understanding of medical ethics provides us with the conceptual wherewithal to find the answers.

To resolve a case or policy question, medical ethicists assume the following four-step process: one to identify the relevant facts and values, two to factor in the probabilities that efforts can realize values, three to prioritize the value of alternative courses of action, and four to make an individual or collective decision regarding the single best course of action available. This is not to say that the decision will be or should be easy or immediate. On the contrary, the issues are complex, and those persons involved with deciding the issue are fallible human beings no matter how intelligent, informed, and morally sensitive they may be. Decision makers may call on different experts from different fields to help decide the issue. Discussions may be contentious and persistent. People often expect that the smoke will dissipate enough so that each individual will come to think that one course of action is better than the alternatives, unless the options are considered morally equal. When enough individuals agree as to which alternative is the best, the issue is considered more or less resolved until someone voices compelling objections. Jonsen, Siegler, and Winslade remain optimistic that they can find which norm should override competing norms for an issue. Interestingly, not all medical ethicists believe that we can find reasons to justify single best answers to questions of ethics and medical ethics.

6. Engelhardt's Postmodern Libertarianism

Engelhardt and I share the view that medical ethics often proceeds without regard to our moral limits. To Engelhardt, the limitations of the Enlightenment project, the attempt to resolve disputes with reason, has contributed to a diversity of moral viewpoints largely ignored by the medical ethics community. In his words:

> Many provide bioethics consultations or advice as if there were one content-full bioethics, one canonical content-full bioethical orthodoxy, that should guide all secular moral decisions and justify all healthcare policy. Such consultants work somewhat as priests, rabbis, or ministers do within a religious context, but without acknowledging their sectarian position .... They speak for reason as such, without acknowledging the particular moral commitments that guide their choices ... there are diverse and profoundly different moral understandings: bioethics is in the plural.[51]

By "secular morality" Engelhardt means an ethic grounded in reason, human nature, or reality itself, instead of a religious or moral tradition.[52] For the purposes of this book, we must understand what Engelhardt means by "content-full bioethics," "secular morality," and "pluralism"; why he believes we have a plurality of moral viewpoints; what pluralism means for those of us engaged in medical ethics.

By "pluralism," Engelhardt refers to diverse moral communities such as the Amish, Orthodox Christians, Roman Catholics, Hindus, or egalitarians, not a plurality of intrinsic values as has been championed by philosophers mentioned in chapter one. Members of a community constitute moral friends in that they function within a framework that provides them with answers to moral questions, or with the means to find answers to moral questions. In this sense the morality of friends is content-full.[53] As Engelhardt says, "Only in terms of the values that direct such communities does one learn which moral and nonmoral goods ought to be pursued and at what costs."[54] By contrast, members of diverse communities constitute moral strangers because they do not share enough moral content to agree as to what would count as an appropriate moral solution to a moral problem.[55] He clarifies:

> People meet as moral strangers when (1) they have different views regarding the morality of a particular endeavor, such as euthanasia, surrogate motherhood, or justice and healthcare, and (2) have no common content-full moral or philosophical framework, which would allow a rational, morally content-full resolution of the controversy at issue.[56]

Engelhardt believes that secular bioethics is a morality of strangers.[57] To resolve moral controversies by rational argument, we must share moral premises, rules of moral inference, and the moral authority to resolve controversies. He specifies part of the problem with reaching moral consensus through rational deliberation as an inability to resolve moral controversies between members of diverse communities and the inability to compare and rank the value of alternative actions. Engelhardt clarifies:

> To judge that some outcomes are better or worse than others, or to judge what people ought to do, one must first rank the major goals of, or moral constraints on, human conduct or devise an algorithm for coordinating or weighting them. In order to justify establishing a particular healthcare system, one will need to decide many matters of policy which presuppose such rankings and algorithms. The difficulty is to justify a particular canonical ranking or account of values. Depending on the priority one assigns to liberty, equality, prosperity, security, and other goals, one will be obliged to endorse radically different social systems, including radically different systems for the distribution of healthcare resources. One can only discover the morally correct social system if one can identify a canonical moral ranking, account, algorithm, or moral sense.[58]

He does not believe that we have a way to discover the correct canonical hierarchy or account. Consider, for example, the difficulty with attempting to resolve the issue over whether we should allow individuals to sell their organs. Engelhardt:

> Nor will it help to appeal to principles of beneficence to determine whether it is morally good or bad for people to sell their organs unless

one already has a common understanding of exploitation, the importance of free choice, the importance of financial advantage, and so on. The advocates of organ sales and the opponents of organ sales often constitute their moral lives within radically different, taken-for-granted moral assumptions. Advocates may see no moral difference between selling their organs and selling their labor, if the risks and returns are comparable. Moreover, advocates may see a nobility in individuals having the freedom and responsibility to make such choices over their own lives.[59]

We may attempt to resolve disputes related to the selling of organs by close attention to details, the application of Beauchamp and Childress's four principles, or the examination of broader intellectual concerns. Engelhardt rejects the view that we can resolve controversies by appealing to mid-level principles such as those advanced by Beauchamp and Childress and shared by different moral theorists. According to Engelhardt, mid-level principles can work for those in the same or similar life worlds but not for those who have different moral perspectives such as Rawlsians and Nozickians. Engelhardt means to highlight differences between Rawlsians who place a greater emphasis on the value of equal opportunity, fraternity, and a more egalitarian distribution of financial resources than do Nozickians, who value individual liberty more highly than Rawlsians. Such differences run deep because individuals may disagree over the existence of inalienable private property rights or the proper ranking of the value of liberty and equality.[60]

Engelhardt believes that attempts to resolve disputes such as those between Rawlsians and Nozickians lead us to seek moral foundations, but he believes this attempt results in either question begging responses or an infinite regress of reasons.[61] With others he declares that the Enlightenment project failed in its quest to find fundamental principles providing singular answers to moral questions. He thinks unyielding controversies illustrate this failure.

Not surprisingly, Engelhardt does not celebrate moral pluralism, but describes the culture of bioethics as a "fragmentation of moral perspective," as a polytheism of perspectives with its chaos of moral diversity, and as a "cacophony of . . . contradictory claims."[62] His view is postmodern in the sense that we face a multiplicity of moral perspectives where disagreements are deep and unyielding.

What are we to do in the face of multiple moral communities and deep disagreements? According to Engelhardt, without justifiable reasons for our moral views, the only escape from nihilism and brute force is agreement among citizens. Engelhardt's view is minimalistic in that it only requires that we respect the freedom of individuals as necessary and sufficient for agreement. He is not celebrating the value of individual autonomy, but demonstrating the minimal conditions of a secular morality in a pluralistic world. Respect for individuals' freedom entails consent to peaceably negotiate. Beyond agreement among citizens, we have no moral justification for our views.

Yet, we must wonder how moral strangers will agree to anything. What sense would it make to adduce a moral reason to a moral stranger? Is it possible that moral strangeness comes in degrees or is a matter of extent? How do we sort out our moral views as members of several communities and organizations? Without answers to these questions, we may be inclined to think that Engelhardt has pushed moral skepticism too far.

Engelhardt does make an effort to escape the quagmire he believes secular bioethics to be. Engelhardt's moral minimalism centers on the principle that we should not infringe upon individuals' freedom. Again, he holds this position not because respecting autonomy is intrinsically valuable, but because he believes it to be the only escape from nihilism, unconstrained relativism, or brute force. From this apparently innocuous idea, he derives the view that the state has no moral justification for infringing upon individuals' freedom and that makes his view in effect libertarian. But we can ask, why should we consent to peaceable negotiation? His answer is prudential in that if we do not agree to peaceably negotiate we lose grounds to object to force used against us. For example, whereas Engelhardt found no moral grounds to defend or oppose people selling their organs, based on his postmodern libertarianism he finds that "people have a secular basic moral right to sell their organs for transplantation."[63]

Although Engelhardt's approach to medical ethics involves a skeptical view of moral knowledge and the ability to resolve disagreements through rational argument, he too has significant similarities with Beauchamp and Childress. Like Beauchamp and Childress, Engelhardt accepts the principles of beneficence and autonomy; only he refers to the principle of autonomy as the principle of permission because he does not wish to imply that autonomy is valuable for the purposes of establishing a basis for secular morality. He also discusses the principle of justice but says that it derives from the principle of beneficence. Engelhardt does not discuss a principle of nonmaleficence, but his comments regarding a duty to forbear from harm entail many of the same consequences as a principle of nonmaleficence. Like Beauchamp and Childress, throughout his text he mentions that principles conflict and that we must weigh conflicting principles to decide what we should do. Although I do not share Engelhardt's moral skepticism, I appreciate his acknowledgment of the problem with ranking the value of alternative actions.

In Part Three I will show how we can appreciate the problem of incommensurability without feeling as if we must choose between nihilism, unconstrained relativism, brute force, or Engelhardt's postmodern libertarianism. More immediately, in chapter two I will take a step toward overcoming Engelhardt's moral skepticism by developing constructive pluralism. For now, I return to Cliff's choice.

7. Cliff's Choice Revisited

Cliff eagerly wishes to donate his only kidney and to go on dialysis. He appears to be rational and his reasons are understandable. Cliff says he is an elderly man with an easy-going lifestyle; he does not believe dialysis would severely diminish his quality of life. Given Russell's medical condition, he might die without Cliff's sacrifice. Recall that physicians ruled out Russell's mother, Eva, on medical grounds in the earlier stages and later considered her as a potential donor only with much hesitation. These may not be all of the relevant facts of the case. After all, the video does not clarify how donating his kidney would affect Cliff's life. Still, we have enough information to understand medical ethics and the dynamics of the case.

In terms of the values of the case, saving Russell's life and protecting Cliff's well-being are beneficent. Retrieving Cliff's kidney would not be a violation of Cliff's autonomy or his right to be free from coercion. Performing the transplant would respect Cliff's choice, fulfill his preferences, and be an expression of his deeply held values, foremost among them, the love he has for Russell. On the other hand, all other things being equal, healthcare providers should not place one patient in peril for the sake of another patient. The hospital should maintain its reputation as a place of healing, and seriously endangering Cliff's life for Russell's is not justifiable. We do not know with certainty whether a transplant would seriously endanger Cliff's life, Eva's life if she donated a kidney, or whether they would find a suitable cadaver kidney for Russell. The question is, do we know enough of the facts and values to know what the transplant team should have done in this case?

The medical details of Cliff's health would help us evaluate the justification of the transplant. Retrieving another kidney from Cliff and subjecting him to dialysis would diminish his quality of life. After all, one reason for performing kidney transplants is that the quality of life of transplant patients is better than the quality of life of patients on dialysis. I have never read an essay on the quality of life of kidney transplant patients compared to the quality of life of dialysis patients that claimed that transplants tend to improve the quality of life of patients except for patients who lead a sedentary lifestyle. Cliff could respond to life on dialysis well enough to live a long life. If the decision not to allow Cliff to donate his only kidney resulted in Russell dying in middle age, many of us would think that they should have performed the transplant. One problem is that we do not know what the outcomes will be.

We could supplement the Beauchamp and Childress model in the hope of resolving the issue. For example, we could focus on a different set of values including loyalty and parental love to help resolve the case. We could try to show how the distinction between directly harming a patient (Cliff) is worse than allowing harm to another patient (Russell). Even if we consider different values and principles, we must still face the conflicts in the case and difficulties with comparing values. An alternative approach to Cliff's choice would not guarantee that we could find a single best course of action to take. Even if an alternative moral approach to Cliff's choice resolves the case better than the Beauchamp and Childress model, there will be cases and policy questions that remain frustratingly difficult and that leave us with much uncertainty. Constructive pluralism acknowledges that such uncertainties and the imprecision of comparing values can obstruct the process of finding the best course of action available. Yet, we are required to make a good decision.

My interpretation is that Cliff made the best choice in donating his kidney to Neil instead of Russell, and that the transplant team at Middlesex Hospital made a *justifiable* decision in refusing to allow Cliff to donate his only kidney to Russell. I am skeptical, though, about whether we can develop a compelling case that the hospital made the *best* decision in refusing to accede to Cliff's preference to donate his remaining kidney. Absent a compelling medical fact to decide the issue, a satisfactory argument would have to address whether Cliff's well-being outweighs the value of satisfying Cliff's preference and Russell's well-being and, perhaps, his life. We would also need a thorough examination of whether the doing versus allowing distinction illuminates a proper action for this case. Doubtless, one could make a serious attempt at developing such an argument. One could also make the case that they should have performed the transplant based on satisfying Cliff's decision and saving Russell's life. Either we accept the view that it was justifiable for the transplant team at Middlesex Hospital to grant or to deny Cliff's decision, or we must be prepared to show why one option deserves priority.

If the transplant team had strong grounds for thinking that it would be better to retrieve a kidney from Eva instead of Cliff, then the case could be resolved in the sense of finding a single best option. Apparently, this was how the case was resolved. I wonder whether the transplant team found additional medical information that tipped the scales in favor of retrieving Eva's kidney or whether they followed a hunch, an intuition, and committed themselves to making the best of that choice. Based on the information in the video, conventional medical ethics underdetermines the answer. In subsequent chapters, I try to show that our beliefs regarding medical ethics are often underdetermined and more tenuous than usually conceived.

On many occasions, a question over what to do about a case or policy will yield a single right answer, a single best alternative we should select. If incommensurability—the inability to sufficiently compare values for the purposes of prioritization—is a commonplace feature of the moral life, we can expect two or more justifiable options regarding how we should decide some cases and policy questions. Once we act on an option, though, we must make the appropriate adjustments to realize value and to avoid or alleviate the fallout of our choices.

In the case of Russell Pendregaust, the efforts of the Pendregaust family and the transplant team at Middlesex Hospital indicate a continuing commitment to Russell and Cliff, what any approach to medical ethics, including constructive pluralism, should entail. The point is that once persons make a choice, those involved with the case are morally required to prevent or alleviate the fallout of the choice. We see from the video that the transplant team at Middlesex Hospital succeeded in this regard. After deciding to refuse to retrieve another kidney from Cliff, the transplant team tried earnestly to find another donor for Russell. If they had retrieved the kidney from Cliff, they then would have been morally required to attend to Cliff's health and quality of life on dialysis, an obvious point that will have more interesting ramifications as we proceed.

8. Conclusion

All of the approaches to medical ethics presented in this chapter contain some merit. We should cultivate virtuous character and relationships; pay attention to contextual details; consider patriarchal influences and abuses of power; and realize our limitations with comparing values. Doubtless, we could examine the approach of other prominent medical ethicists and sharpen our understanding of the similarities and differences among them. What we find in the United States though is a dominant model of thinking about medical ethics characterized by a plurality of moral principles, a belief that principles frequently conflict, and the conviction that we must weigh our alternatives. I invite any doubters of the claim of a dominant model of American medical ethics to peruse the medical ethics literature, especially that written by healthcare providers. I do not pretend to know all of the significant views among medical ethicists, but some of the differences relate to the number of principles they identify and their level of moral skepticism.

Beauchamp and Childress believe that cases can be reasonably resolved, but they present ethics as a revisable body of beliefs. Interestingly, although many within the American medical ethics community accept their four principles, few appreciate their views on the revision of beliefs. When we apply these values and their corresponding principles to Cliff's choice, no answer as to whether the transplant team made the best decision emerges. This conclusion may not surprise Beauchamp and Childress, but it does run counter to conventional medical ethics in the United States heavily influenced by their work. Engelhardt embraces a deeper level of moral skepticism and offers a minimalist morality based on peaceable agreement, but I suspect his views are too skeptical for many medical ethicists. Although I am less skeptical than Engelhardt, we should appreciate some level of moral skepticism. Neither the skeptical elements of Beauchamp and Childress and Engelhardt nor their view that ethics is an evolving process has found its way into mainstream medical ethics.

The failure of many medical ethicists to appreciate our moral limits stems from many sources, but it probably has something to do with commentators not knowing how such views apply to medical ethics or believing that such views are likely to be more destructive than constructive. Another reason may be that Beauchamp and Childress do not discuss the revisability of moral beliefs in much detail or the limitations of ethical decision-making in terms of finding answers for cases or policies. This is a significant qualification, for scholars have criticized their reliance on principles and discussed the relativity of values, usually in terms of how people of different cultures or subcultures have different values. This point about the relativity of values appears to be exactly what Beauchamp and Childress mean by their skepticism toward universal theories. What appears to surprise no one is that this skepticism does not apply to decisions that we must make about cases or policies. Too many commentators remain wildly optimistic that sensitivity to contexts affords us the opportunity to discover unique answers to questions about cases and policies. One only has to peruse the medical ethics literature to see that this is so.

In Part Two of this book, I show that participants to ethical debates related to organ retrieval believe that we can find unique answers with close attention to the relevant values and facts. Throughout this book, I argue that the ethical problems of organ retrieval indicate that we do not always have the moral methods and concepts to find a single best answer. After all, why should we think that each culture or subculture has all of the needed moral concepts for all moral questions for all of its members even if the culture is homogenous based on several criteria? This conclusion need not leave us disappointed with the resources of ethics. Moral beliefs provide us with a system of discourse, meaning, justification, faith, and concepts that guide us in developing a better world. The instability of our beliefs provides us with the opportunity to develop better views of ethics to more effectively address the conflicts thrust upon us by the nature of the world, the flaws in our institutions and concepts, and our individual frailties. In essence, the conflicted world and the ambiguous success of our concepts provide the way for a view of ethics that expects and encourages the improvement of our concepts, institutions, technologies, and development of individual talent and goodness. It encourages us sometimes to shift our thinking from making the best choice to doing well with a good choice.

That Beauchamp and Childress emphasize the fallibility of our theories and judgments and that they regard the moral life as evolving is interesting and helpful. This is precisely the spirit with which I develop constructive pluralism, only I emphasize what they gloss over and I defend unconventional views that they do not appear to accept even though constructive pluralism is consistent with their skeptical remarks. While Beauchamp and Childress mention the revisability of our moral beliefs, I demonstrate how this revision of moral beliefs might develop in the context of organ retrieval. I do this by showing that their claim that we will never develop a completely stable equilibrium between our theories, principles, and judgments is vastly understated.

What I show in the chapters on treating the dead with proper moral regard, defining death, xenotransplantation, selling organs, and stem cell research is that our moral views of cases, practices, policies, and theories are more tenuous than typically conceived by medical ethicists. Widely shared views relevant to the field of medical ethics partially consist of hopes, vague intuitions, superstitions, and flimsy justifications that frequently lead to counter intuitive results. Since I believe many of our moral limits stem from the incommensurability of values, I discuss the need to revise our beliefs in the light of difficulties with weighing or ranking the value of our options.

Engelhardt and I share skepticism about comparisons of value, but while he bases morality on an agreement among citizens, I develop constructive pluralism that emphasizes morality as a continual constructive process. Interestingly, Engelhardt uses a building metaphor to describe morality, but he does not develop the idea. In his words, "From a general secular perspective, one might consider the different moral communities as experiments in the building of moral worlds, as creative endeavors to fashion views of the good life and alternative content-full bioethics."[64] This is precisely what I aim to do with constructive pluralism. In the next chapter, I demonstrate the need for constructive pluralism by defending the view that some of our options are incommensurable and that the weighing metaphor helps us to understand the limitations of our moral intuitions.

Three

PLURALISM, INCOMMENSURABILITY, AND WEIGHING

I have presented a view of the moral life in which a plurality of moral values often conflict. When we face a moral conflict, we need to determine whether an option is obligatory, permissible, or supererogatory. Frequently, we need to determine whether one option has more overall value than alternative options or whether the options appear to have equal value. To make such determinations, the value of the options must be comparable in some significant way, significant enough to justify our choices. As we have seen, scholars frequently utilize the weighing metaphor to show that one option is better, that it outweighs alternatives. We have also seen that Hugo Tristram Engelhardt believes that we lack justifiable foundations for our value comparisons. In this chapter, I attempt to clarify the meaning of moral pluralism, the meaning of incommensurability, show why some options are incommensurable, and demonstrate the efficacy and limitations of the weighing metaphor.

1. Moral Pluralism

We have seen that different moral philosophers believe in a plurality of intrinsic goods, but that they often disagree as to the number and nature of those goods. I also argued that our subjective experiences of value, the phenomenology of value, means that we experience value as a plurality of goods. Pluralism about the good is often thought to contrast with utilitarianism and Kantian deontology that state moral judgments can be reduced to a single value or principle: for utilitarians, the value may be pleasure, happiness, or preference satisfaction, and for Kantians, respect for persons as ends in themselves.[1]

Others have attempted to reconcile pluralism with Kantianism and utilitariansism. Peter Railton concedes that orthodox Kantians may not be able to accommodate pluralism, but argues that the core of Kantian ethics can become pluralistic by broadening Kant's moral psychology to include benevolent feelings along with reason as moral bases for action.[2] We accomplish this reconciliation by noting that reflection, insight, and self-control shape or change our feelings, thereby leaving persons with complex admixtures of reason and feeling as moral motives. For Railton, benevolence is more like a skill whose exercise is often spontaneous, but its acquisition and cultivation require deliberation. Railton means that impulsive acts of benevolence do not exemplify autonomy in Kant's sense, but the conscious cultivation of other-regarding sentiments that then form the bases of benevolent actions are indirectly autonomous.

The attempt to reconcile pluralism with utilitarianism meets with less controversy. John Stuart Mill argued for different types of pleasures—intellectual and sensual, and that many goods constitute happiness.[3] Recently, Brad Hooker has offered a version of rule consequentialism in which two values, fairness and well-being, form the basis of selecting moral rules.[4] Hooker claims that well-being consists in a plurality of goods including pleasure, friendship, and achievement.[5] In the light of pluralism's association with diverse venerable philosophical traditions, Lawrence Becker claims that "all significant moral theories appear to be pluralistic at one level or another."[6] This may be an overstatement, but many ethical theorists offer pluralistic accounts of intrinsic goodness.

As a theory of right action, pluralism implies situations in which no single correct moral answer is possible. Susan Wolf characterizes areas of moral indeterminacy as having more than one right answer, or as having no right answer.[7] According to pluralists about right action, responses to a moral problem may justifiably diverge due to cultural or individual differences, or from incommensurable features constitutive of moral conflicts.[8] This is not to say that pluralists view themselves as repackaging the same cultural relativism or subjectivism. Wolf believes pluralism offers a path between relativism that denies any unique moral answers exist, and a kind of absolutism that entails single right answers for all cases, but pluralism suggest some moral problems have unique answers, other problems do not.[9]

Although John Kekes believes conflicts among values must be resolved within cultural traditions, he claims some values, primary values, such as food, shelter, and a sense of belonging are cross-cultural.[10] For Kekes, no value is always overriding, and so different cultural conditions may yield different rational results when values conflict.[11] Each of these three pluralist approaches deserves further explication.

Pluralists such as Kekes and Wolf give cultural traditions a key role in resolving moral conflicts. Kekes claims that the best action will be the one that maintains our common system of values.[12] I suspect that what Kekes has in mind is that a culture such as the United States that celebrates individual liberty, liberty will carry much weight in times of conflict with other values such as the public good. What this means for concrete moral controversies remains foggy. For instance, both a market economy and an altruistic tradition of organ donation exist concurrently. On Kekes's view, how are we to decide whether we should permit the selling of organs? Even if we can give a unique answer to this question, we must wonder if all countries should prohibit or permit the selling of organs. Although Kekes distinguishes his brand of pluralism from cultural relativism, by relativizing rational conflict resolution to culture, Kekes must accept the view that different cultures may justifiably respond to an issue differently. In this way, Kekes must believe that some moral problems do not admit of unique solutions. Perhaps Kekes believes in unique rational responses to moral conflicts within a culture. Unfortunately, for the clarification and development of moral pluralism, Kekes does not address the resolution of concrete cases of conflicting values. Consequently, it remains unclear how Kekes could offer guidance when attempting to resolve moral conflicts in applied ethics such as those related to organ retrieval.

Wolf also emphasizes the role of culture in determining moral responses to conflicting values. She adds that persons' appropriate responses depend upon their identification with a culture or subculture.[13] Wolf contends that different actions can both be justifiable depending on the overall self-concept of the persons facing a conflict.[14] She has us imagine, for example, two persons, one Amish the other a police detective, wondering how to respond to an aggressive person bent on striking them. The violent person creates a conflict between the value of keeping the peace with the value of being free from harm. According to Wolf, it may be right for the Amish person to remain a pacifist while the detective can utilize force in self-defense. Significantly, being a member of a culture does not always require one to behave in a unique way: she leaves it open that persons can justifiably choose whether to remain a member.

How are persons to respond to conflicts when contemplating their sense of self? Elizabeth Anderson answers this question by claiming that emphasizing the role of a person's narrative unity can resolve some conflicts. In broad terms, I take this to mean that individuals should tell a story that provides him or her a sense of who he or she is, how he or she arrived there, and how he or she wants to develop for the future. However true, this process does not necessarily reveal what people should do, especially when a large part of American discourse encourages individuals to reinvent themselves. The implications of this for Anderson's view remain unclear, but Kekes and Wolf suggest that for each person facing a conflict, a single correct response usually exists.

Michael Stocker, on the other hand, contemplates a person considering whether to take the bus or car across town.[15] I do not consider this a moral conflict, but this example involves a conflict of values that can be illustrative. The bus is cheaper and obviates the need to find a parking space, but the car is quicker and more convenient in terms of allowing the person to leave whenever the person pleases. The decision requires considering many values such as pleasantness, time, and the freedom and ease that money brings. Doubtless further details will give guidance, but Stocker believes, correctly, that either option is permissible. Stocker's example shows the interesting thesis that value conflicts can yield several justifiable responses for persons in the same circumstances. The possibility of right action for persons in the same circumstances stands in contrast with venerable views of moral philosophy, including the philosophy of prominent moral pluralists.

The impulse to identify right action, even in the face of conflicting values, with justified unique responses is strong. That we wonder which of conflicting moral opinions is true suggests a right answer exists, presumably a unique answer that we can and should discover. It makes sense to wonder which action is best, instead of merely what is good. Not surprisingly, some pluralists believe moral questions have single answers. William David Ross believed that we are to apprehend the right action through rational intuition.[16]

Thomas Nagel believes that even if we accept the view that a plurality of values often conflict, we can still find unique solutions. For Nagel, good judgment steps in where good theory leaves off. In his words, "our capacity to resolve conflicts in particular cases may extend beyond our capacity to enunciate general principles that explain those resolutions."[17] Interestingly, many pluralists while willing to accept a plurality of goods often attempt to unify right action. Or even when they accept a plurality of right action, they relativize correct action to a culture or subject. We saw this with the philosophy of contemporary pluralists such as Wolf, Kekes, and Anderson. I believe that the scope of the plurality of right action is greater than many suppose due to the incommensurability of values.

Pluralism in terms of right action contrasts with traditional utilitarianism and deontological theories of right action. Take hedonistic act utilitarianism, for example. Pleasure is the sole good, and right action is that which maximizes pleasure for each moral decision. For hedonistic act utilitarians, there will be a unique right response for each moral decision unless different actions produce equal amounts of pleasure. In those cases, persons may as well flip a coin as to which possible act to choose; either option is right. Immanuel Kant allows for a plurality of right action only in cases of imperfect duties. For example, we have an imperfect duty to be benevolent, because we can satisfy this requirement in many ways.[18] Kant is also notorious for arguing that in the case of perfect duties, contextual details do not alter our duties. So, in the case of perfect duties, there can be no plurality of right action. Aristotle also talks about hitting a moral target when we deliberate; he does not discuss moral targets for moral decisions.[19]

The plurality of right action results from the inability to adequately compare some of our options and that choosing well is justification enough for many moral choices. What we need is a better understanding and defense of the incommensurability of some moral choices.

2. Incommensurability

Not all philosophers define "incommensurability" in the same way, but the debate over incommensurable values is whether we can justify choosing one alternative instead of another in a case based on a comparison of the moral values involved. Those inclined to think some choices involve incommensurable values must wonder why the alternatives are not sufficiently comparable. Some philosophers believe values are incommensurable because no common scale to measure or weigh the values exists. Often, philosophers explain the absence of a common scale to evaluate alternatives as a function of value pluralism. The idea is that values are different and so no single scale can measure or weigh them. Some philosophers believe, for instance, that a deontological value such as respect for persons and the utilitarian value of maximizing happiness do not reduce to the same scale.[20] On some accounts the absence of a common scale defines incommensurability. Ruth Chang defines incommensurable values as involving alternatives that resist measurement by a common scale of units of value.[21]

On other accounts, the incommensurability of values means that we cannot compare values in the sense of being able to assign an authoritative ordinal or cardinal ranking.[22] With an ordinal ranking of values we can list the value of alternatives in a hierarchical order; a cardinal ranking means that we can numerically rank the value of alternatives in accordance with some unit of value.[23] A strong version of incommensurability means that we cannot give a cardinal or an ordinal ranking to competing values. Incommensurable values in the strong sense leave us without a means of appropriately giving different values precise rankings, say 5 versus 3, or of ranking one value higher or equal to another.[24] We say values are incommensurable in the strong sense if and only if we cannot rationally state one alternative to be better, worse, or equal to another.[25] Chang calls this view of incommensurability the trichotomy thesis because values have three possible priority relations.

Chang introduces a fourth relation between values; values can be on a par.[26] Anderson explains that values would be on a par if, for example, we could justify saying that a novel is as good a novel as a painting is a good painting.[27] While it may make sense to consider whether values are on a par in some contexts, this may not be helpful in comparing conflicting values regarding organ retrieval. I doubt that it would be helpful to wonder whether a heart transplant is as good a heart transplant as a liver transplant is a liver transplant or whether a treatment regimen for failing kidneys is as good at treating kidneys as a treatment for AIDS is for treating AIDS.

Terrance McConnell believes commensurability comes in degrees because some comparative judgments between deontological and consequentialist values are possible even if they cannot be reduced to a common scale.[28] For instance, breaking small promises (presumably a deontological violation) can be justified for the sake of saving lives (presumably a consequentialist value).[29] McConnell's example is unsatisfactory, because breaking small promises can have morally relevant consequences and saving lives can have deontological value. But his point is understandable and his judgment about promise breaking and saving lives is justified.

Why McConnell regards this example as showing that commensurability can come in degrees is not obvious. McConnell could say that breaking small promises is less of a deontological evil than allowing people to die is a consequentialist evil. If this description of the comparison were correct, we would have an obvious application of Chang's concept of values on a par. Still, we would need some criteria for making cross-scale comparisons and reasons for understanding how cross-scale comparisons render commensurability as a matter of degree. Without identifying the moral criteria for making such judgments, why should we believe that commensurability comes in degrees? After all, it could be that we have intuitively grasped a common scale to compare deontological and consequentialist values but have failed to articulate the nature of the scale.

Even if conceiving of commensurability in terms of degrees makes sense when defined in terms of having a common scale by which to prioritize values, it does not make sense when we define commensurability in terms of the trichotomy thesis. Predicates such as "better than" and "worse than" come in degrees, but this does not mean that commensurability comes in degrees. It does mean that goodness and badness can come in degrees, and it remains significant to think of degrees of goodness and badness for the sake of comparing the value of organ retrieval strategies.

I will dispense with the idea of degrees of incommensurability. Whether values are commensurable is an either/or proposition. Since I see no obvious application of regarding values on a par, I will also define incommensurability in terms of the trichotomy thesis. That is, I am interested in whether we can determine an option to be better than, equal to, or less than another option with respect to its overall value. Whenever I refer to "commensurability," I mean we can justifiably prioritize the value of options.

Most philosophers do not believe that all values are incommensurable or that no values are incommensurable. James Griffin believes philosophers have overestimated the frequency of cases involving incommensurable values.[30] Along this line, Ray Gillespie Frey believes that widespread incommensurability is at odds with the moral decisions that we actually make.[31] Frey also thinks that value conflicts can be rationally resolved if and only if we can compare values. If Frey is right, most of our moral decisions involve commensurable values or are non-rational resolutions. Although commentators often omit to clarify what they mean by "rational resolution," I suspect they mean that a clash of values is rationally resolved if and only if a unique response is justified, or if reason shows that different responses are permissible. Since Frey is unwilling to accept the conclusion that most of our moral decisions are non-rational, he finds it reasonable to believe that most value conflicts involve commensurable values. For Frey, whether values are incommensurable has great practical import.

I have already stated that I believe some value conflicts involve incommensurable values. Chang and Donald Regan have developed interesting arguments against the belief in incommensurable values. I defend the incommensurability of values while acknowledging the strength of some of Chang and Regan's arguments.

3. Covering Values

A core premise for understanding Chang's views on incommensurability pertains to her concept of a covering value. She defines "covering value" as "any consideration with respect to which a meaningful comparison can be made."[33] According to Chang, asking questions such as whether philosophy is better than pushpin is not sensible without identifying the respect to which we compare philosophy with pushpin. She says that philosophy may be better with respect to understanding intrinsic worthwhileness but pushpin may be better for relaxation or hand-eye coordination.[34] On her view, only with respect to covering values are comparisons intelligible.

With the concept of a covering value in mind, Chang clarifies that we need to disambiguate what we mean in saying two options are incomparable, or to use my preferred term, incommensurable. It could mean no covering value with which to compare two options exists or that two options are incomparable with respect to an identified covering value.[35] With organ retrieval, the second conception of incomparability is often relevant. We may identify the end of the problem of premature or congenital organ failure as a covering value, but not be able to compare whether stem cell research or xenotransplantation is the best means of realizing that value.

Yet, we cannot characterize all comparisons within the framework of covering values. We may agree that rejecting the dead donor rule better satisfies the value of retrieving more transplantable organs and that such a move does not satisfy the value of respecting human life, but we may be at a loss as to whether we should reject the dead donor rule. When we consider a society that prohibits killing persons for their organs, and another society that rejects the dead donor rule, the overall value of living in those societies all other things remaining equal is what we are attempting to grasp. For this reason, Chang's good point about identifying covering values does not apply to all comparisons that we need to make.

My disagreement with Chang influences the way in which I evaluate some of her arguments against incommensurability, but not always. In what follows, I will consider six issues related to incommensurability: the plurality of values, the calculation of values, the irresolvability of conflict, the multiple ranking of values, the argument from small improvements, and the argument from improved education and skill. These issues do not exhaust the concerns of Chang and Regan, but they do address what I perceive as the most interesting arguments against the presence of incommensurable value conflicts.

4. The Plurality of Values

For Chang, the commonality among arguments of this type is that a difference between two items can be great enough to preclude a basis of comparison. Chang notes that the argument from the diversity of values may come in many forms, depending on whether the differences in value allegedly stem from being different types of value, different dimensions or scales of value, or different genres.[36] I prefer the term "plurality" over "diversity" for the sake of consistency with the rest of this book. We can understand "plurality of values" and the argument from the "plurality of values" in many ways as shown by different thinkers such as Ross, Stocker, and Engelhardt.

This argument entails that values are incommensurable in principle, some values are impossible to compare based on their intrinsic differences. Chang attempts to undermine this argument with a strategy she calls the nominal-notable test. She invites us to compare the value of Mozart's creativity with the value of Michelangelo's creativity.[37] For those inclined to think that Wolfgang Amadeus Mozart's creativity is incomparable to Michelangelo Buonarroti's creativity because their activities are different, she asks us to compare the creative value of a painter of little talent with Mozart's creative value. Obviously, Mozart's creative value is better than the creative value of the painter with little talent. Her point is that even though Mozart expressed his creativity differently from that of the nominal painter, we can make a justified comparison that Mozart has greater creative value. To her mind, whatever makes it difficult to compare Mozart's creative value with Michelangelo's creative value cannot be due to plural values underlying or constituting different activities.

Chang's argument does not adequately address the sorts of comparative questions we must often ask. Chang goes too far by first assuming that trying to compare the overall value of an item is not sensible. For example, we may legitimately wonder whether leading a life as a competent but unremarkable surgeon is better than leading a life as a remarkable but financially poor artist. Undergraduates must ask themselves these sorts of questions before declaring a major area of study. Wealth is not the only value they need to compare. They need to consider the overall value of two different careers and lifestyles.

As we attempt to understand an undergraduate's career choice, details will help us appraise which life is better for that individual. It will be crucial to understand the individual's attitude toward poverty, wealth, medicine, and art. An individual's psychological profile can leave us in a quandary as to what would be the better life for that individual. For this reason, the individual contemplating the decision may be unable to determine the best life or decide to make the most of a decision.

Similarly, comparing the value of organ retrieval strategies is difficult in part because one strategy may be more successful than another strategy at retrieving more organs but less successful in honoring another value such as the respect for life. Xenotransplants, for example, may someday save the lives of many humans but only at the expense of pigs. Likewise, redefining death according to the higher brain definition may allow for the retrieval of more organs, but at the risk of taking organs from people who may still be alive. Making these sorts of comparisons is difficult and the values involved may be incommensurable. The incommensurability of some decisions is due in part to the differences in the types of values involved. If we were only considering the value of organ retrieval strategies in terms of their potential for saving human life, our value comparisons would be easier although still difficult. We must consider the overall value of each organ retrieval strategy. If "overall value" sounds too mystical, then we are merely attempting to compare the value of options by considering all of the relevant moral factors. Even if we follow Chang's advice in identifying a covering value, we will invariably have multiple covering values to consider.

5. The Calculation of Values

The argument regarding calculations rests upon the view that if values are commensurable, then they must contain the same basic unit of value amenable to quantitative analysis in terms of addition and subtraction. Anderson rejects the view that we can quantitatively analyze values based on examples of comparing the value of friendship with the life of one's mother.[38] If Anderson is correct, then either some values are incommensurable or commensurability does not entail that all values are calculable.

Chang believes that we can compare the value of different options without presupposing that we can add and subtract values. She claims that we can determine the manner in which or the extent to which one option is more valuable than another option without implying that the values consist of the same units. She also claims that the value of some options, such as the number of lives saved, is open to quantification.[39]

To appreciate Chang's point, we need to keep in mind that only three options have the potential to seriously address the problem of premature organ failure: a full-scale preventive medicine campaign, xenotransplantation, and stem cell research. Successful preventive medicine will not eliminate the need for organ transplantation, but many diseases that ravage human organs are preventable. Xenotransplantation has the potential to extend the lives of many thousands of heart and kidney transplant patients, but only at the expense of animals' lives. Stem cell research has the greatest potential for saving lives, but is controversial for its research based on embryos and fetuses. In chapter nine I will discuss evidence suggesting that adult stem cells can develop into different tissues. Adult stem cell research then has the greatest potential to save lives without violating other values. We can accept this conclusion without claiming that comparing the value of organ retrieval strategies will always be possible with our current level of moral and medical knowledge.

6. The Irresolvability of Conflict

The first chapter highlighted difficulties with resolving moral conflict. Since some moral conflicts appear irresolvable in the sense that they defy our efforts to find a single best response, it appears that some values are incommensurable. Chang rejects this argument for two reasons. To understand the debate over the irresolvability of moral conflict and the implications for incommensurability, it helps to distinguish between incommensurability in principle and incommensurability in fact.

Incommensurability in principle is the view that precludes the possibility of adequately comparing options for the purposes of ranking their value. This view entails that reality prevents us from adequately comparing values for the purposes of choice. Such comparisons are not possible any more than making two and two equal five. Incommensurability in principle is what Griffin has in mind when he says, "we have uncovered incommensurability not when we cannot decide how to rank values but when we can decide that they are unrankable."[40] Incommensurability in fact is the view that with our current level of moral understanding we cannot adequately compare options for the sake of ranking their value. The view states that given our current state of knowledge, we cannot compare values adequately enough to show that one option is better than, worse than, or equal to another option.

The first of Chang's reasons for rejecting the argument from the irresolvability of conflict pertains to incommensurability in principle. Chang states that this argument presupposes verificationism; a view of truth stemming from early twentieth century philosophy of science.[41] Verificationism is the view that all semantically meaningful statements are verifiable as true. According to verificationists, unverifiable statements are nonsensical. A statement such as "Saturday is red" is nonsensical even though the statement is grammatically correct because no conditions could support its truth.

Despite the initial appeal of verificationism, it has been widely rejected, largely because many statements are obviously semantically meaningful even though we may never know whether the statement is true or false. For example, we can say that the famous heart surgeon Denton Cooley studied for eight hours on 8 August 1972. Most of us do not know whether this statement is true or even how to determine its truth-value, but the statement is not nonsensical. I do not intend to attempt to rehabilitate verificationism. I agree with

Chang about the argument from the irresolvability of conflict as it applies to incommensurability in principle.

Chang's second reason for rejecting the argument from the irresolvability of conflict addresses my concern over whether a conflict is incommensurable in fact. She states that we cannot always know whether a conflict is irresolvable and whether we have exhausted all of the value relations between two options.[42] But conflict can be difficult to resolve without being incommensurable. The persistence of irresolvability can lend inductive support to thinking that the conflict is irresolvable. Even if the conflict is potentially commensurable and resolvable, if it escapes our current level of understanding, we are still stuck with the problem of deciding what we should do in the light of the irresolvable conflict. After we seriously reflect on the comparative value of two options utilizing the best that moral philosophy and common sense have to offer and fail to resolve disagreement, the options are incommensurable in fact. Although prominent philosophers such as Chang and Griffin concentrate on the ontological thesis, incommensurability in fact is a significant issue as well. In chapter eleven, I will demonstrate in my development of constructive pluralism that incommensurability in fact leads to interesting results for both ethics and applied ethics.

7. Education and Skill

In contrast to most philosophers, Regan defends the view that we are unjustified in thinking that any values are incommensurable.[43] Regan acknowledges the practical difficulty of determining which of two options has the greater value, but he also notes that education and refined skill can improve a person's ability to make accurate comparisons. He realizes that incommensurability in principle does not follow from incommensurability in fact. As we develop our knowledge, we become better equipped to make value comparisons. What appears incommensurable at first glance may be commensurable after we learn more about the subject matter. As we gain knowledge about different organ retrieval strategies, we will be in a better position to make value comparisons regarding organ retrieval. For these reasons, Regan suggests that we are not justified in rejecting the possibility of successfully comparing the value of all alternative options. Even if we cannot make accurate value comparisons individually or collectively, it remains theoretically possible that we can discover an accurate value comparison. Even if we do not presently know how the values of two alternatives compare, it does not mean that a true or accurate comparison is impossible.

Even if Regan is right that all value comparisons are commensurable in theory, we must still face practical circumstances where we do not know which conflicting alternative ranks higher or whether the options are equal in value. Regan's view appears true, but we should note that specialists often

disagree about which organ retrieval strategies are more moral. These disagreements often result from different value comparisons. We need to better
understand why this is so and what we should do when we find ourselves in
such circumstances. I offer a practical argument in defense of the incommensurability of values that draws on an analogy between making value comparisons and weighing objects. As we have seen, much of the discussion of
comparing values utilizes the weighing metaphor. An analysis of the weighing
metaphor clarifies the nature of some moral disagreements, the prospects and
limits of our moral knowledge, and the nature of leading moral lives. In turn,
this moral understanding sheds light on debates related to organ retrieval.

8. Weighing Our Options

The weighing metaphor is a dominant metaphor in ethics and medical ethics
regarding the resolution of moral conflicts. Tom Beauchamp and James Childress, Albert R. Jonsen, Mark Siegler, William J. Winslade, and H. Tristram
Engelhardt believe that weighing our options must be part of good decisions
in medical contexts. Philosophers of moral theory also utilize the weighing
metaphor. Griffin, for example, says:

> if moral norms are to be comparable across their range, we need an over-
> arching framework, comparable to the notion of the "quality of life" to
> which the various prudential values could all be seen as contributing—
> perhaps the notion of "morality" itself, which might allow all norms to be
> ranked as to their moral "weight" of "importance" or "stringency."[44]

Anderson says that according to the view that we can measure values on the
same scale, "the sole practical role of the concept of value is to assign weights
to goods, so that reason can choose what is weightiest or most valuable."[45] In
describing the merits of his view of moral pluralism, Stocker says that his pluralism "can pose all the problems of plurality that have worried philosophers—preeminently, worries about having to weigh and combine different
evaluative considerations."[46] Many more examples exist of leading moral philosophers and medical ethicists who utilize the weighing metaphor; this suf-
fices as a representative sample. In what follows I show the merits and limitations of the weighing metaphor.

We know that an ordinary pencil weighs less than an ordinary dictionary
without knowing the precise weight of the pencil or the dictionary and without placing the objects on a scale. Experience provides this knowledge when
we lift the objects. We know which is heavier through our muscles, bones,
and nerves. For many objects, we can determine which of two objects is the
heaviest in the same way. In many contexts, we have a type of bodily knowledge, an intuition if you will, of the weights of many objects in terms of being

able to rank them from the heaviest to the lightest. Such judgments are not controversial, and a person's cultural or personal background is irrelevant in determining a ranking of objects from heaviest to lightest. Libertarians, communists, anarchists, fascists, men, women, children, heterosexuals, homosexuals, bisexuals, blacks, whites, Asians, Mexicans, Europeans, Americans, Middle Easterners, Catholics, Buddhists, atheists, and so forth, can agree on the correct ranking of the weights of objects.

We can also be justified in ranking the weights of objects without picking them up. If we rank the weights of an adult elephant, cow, dog, and mouse from the lightest to the heaviest, we know the answer without attempting to lift each animal. Nor do we need to place the animals on a scale. Our experiences justify our judgments. If pressed, we could supply reasons based on our observations of the behavior of each animal, readings about the animals, and so forth. In short, our beliefs about the animals' weights must cohere with a broader body of knowledge. Again, such judgments regarding the relative weights of these animals are not controversial, not even cross-culturally.

In many cases, the weights of two different objects are sufficiently close such that we cannot tell which one is heavier by lifting the objects. In these cases, our intuitive powers about which object is heavier has limitations, and we may not have an intuition as to which object is heavier. If we do have an intuition about ranking the weight of different objects in these close cases, the intuition might be untrustworthy and mistaken. Where objects are close in weight, our ethnicity, religion, nationality, gender, or sexual orientation will not be relevant in helping us determine a proper ranking of objects. It may be the case that a person's occupation or biology can enable the person to be a more accurate judge. A postal worker or grocer might be better in determining a correct ranking of objects' weights than medical ethicists.

In a case where our intuition leaves us with an indeterminate answer to the question as to which of two objects is heavier, we have the option of weighing the objects on a scale to gain the requisite knowledge. In this case, the results of weighing the objects provide a good reason to think that we have a correct ranking of the objects' weights and replaces or supports whatever intuitions a person might have about the initial ranking. This observation supports Beauchamp and Childress's view that we should attempt to replace intuitions with good reasons. In some cases, the objects will be so close in weight that we will not be able to tell which object is heavier even after placing them on a properly functioning scale. In such a case, we can say that the objects weigh the same for practical purposes, unless we need to find a more sensitive scale to determine the heavier of the two objects. A more sensitive scale provides analogous support to Regan's claim that we can develop more skill related to comparing values. In principle, we can develop a more sensitive scale to weigh any two objects, but for many purposes, we only need a close approximation as to an object's weight relative to that of another object.

The weighing metaphor suggests that with some decisions we know the answer as to which action overall is more morally valuable. For example, we know that killing a healthy person for the person's body parts is wrong. The disvalue of killing the healthy person outweighs the value of benefiting a transplant recipient or several transplant recipients. However possible that some horrendous circumstances might convince us killing a healthy person for his or her body parts is sometimes permissible, my underlying point still stands: we know which option carries the most moral weight in some cases.

The existence of organ transplantation demonstrates this truth. As will be shown in chapter four, the value of extending a person's life often outweighs the disvalue of post-operative pain and suffering. These considerations undermine Engelhardt's skepticism. We can be confident that some moral judgments are true and that these judgments are cross-cultural. The skepticism that we have no good grounds for claims to moral knowledge conflicts with the use of the weighing metaphor. We do not always have to find moral foundations to be justified in our moral beliefs.

In cases where answers to moral questions are more difficult, increased knowledge and attention to ethics and medicine can enable us to make better judgments. Individual medical ethicists can better judge the value of organ retrieval strategies when they immerse themselves in the relevant literature. Medical ethicists from different academic backgrounds can better judge the overall value of organ retrieval strategies than those who do not study ethics, medical ethics, medicine, law, religion, medical sociology, or some other relevant field. In some cases, medical ethicists and non-medical ethicists will have difficulty forming an opinion, and there will be considerable disagreement among citizens even after they have studied the relevant issues.

Just as we cannot always tell which of two objects is heavier by lifting the objects or by making an educated guess, we cannot always determine the answer to a moral question. Further reflection may not yield a satisfactory answer either. We cannot expect our moral intuitions or moral reasoning to always give us satisfactory answers when we are trying to weigh the value of conflicting alternatives. As our intuition as to which object is heavier has limitations, so does our intuition about the heavier moral weight of alternatives.

Individuals' cultural or personal background may lead them to have different intuitions. Recall Jonsen, Siegler, and Winslade's example of how Navaho Indians do not always value the disclosure of risks as highly as individuals from other cultures. Scientists and transplant surgeons probably value the acquisition of knowledge and personal achievement more than most laypersons. They also probably value medical progress more than most citizens. Not surprisingly, they expect society to support or tolerate risky medical ventures like xenotransplantation.

Those who have benefited from capitalist economies or who come from an oppressive country or family may place greater value on individual liberty, thereby predisposing them to support markets for organs. Conversely, persons who have experienced or witnessed capitalist exploitation may be more suspicious about a market for organs. Those who have had loved ones die while waiting for an organ transplant will probably value saving transplant patients' lives more than those who have not suffered such a loss. Persons victimized by discrimination or exploitation by a member or organization of a healthcare group may be less inclined to support biomedical research.

For these reasons, all persons involved with organ transplantation should share their perspectives on different organ retrieval strategies and discuss the potential gains and losses of implementing those strategies. Personal experience can sensitize individuals to values, but blind them to potential moral losses of implementing organ retrieval strategies.

Individuals sharing information and experiences about organ retrieval pave the way for understanding and agreement on the policies, practices, and laws we should adopt. If individuals still disagree after these communications, then we risk an impasse and stubborn opposition. Such disagreement also reveals a problem when analogizing the comparison of physical weights with the comparison of moral weights: we do not have a moral analogue to a scale that can determine which of two objects is heavier when our intuitions and reasons about moral weights reach their apparent limit. We are not able to develop moral sensitivity to resolve many disagreements or uncertainties in the way that a more sensitive scale can settle a question about which of two objects is heavier. Education, art, experience, and witnessing the experiences of others can make us more sensitive about the value of an individual or a course of action. This is precisely what organ donor education campaigns attempt to do. Even so, after we present the relevant facts, values, and probabilities, if parties to the discussion still disagree as to what is moral, we have no moral scale to which to appeal. Agreement on moral matters is no assurance that we have properly weighed the moral value of alternatives. To this extent, we can appreciate Engelhardt's skepticism, and for this reason, the lack of a common scale is significant for thinking about incommensurability. Use of the weighing metaphor helps us understand the reasonableness of believing that some values are incommensurable in fact.

At the same time, the weighing metaphor fails to help us evaluate alternative courses of action. The weighing metaphor entices us to regard values as fixed entities open to evaluation at a given time. The problem with utilizing the weighing metaphor for many of the conflicts with organ retrieval is that organ retrieval strategies involve constant transformation. Weighing the moral value of organ retrieval strategies is like trying to weigh objects in the midst of transformation without knowing what the final objects will be like. For this reason, the weighing metaphor is misleading for suggesting that we can add and subtract values and disvalues thereby allowing us to maximize the value of our choices if we calculate the values correctly. The weighing metaphor also fails to capture the dynamic nature of the moral life. With organ retrieval, we are not working with precisely defined values with a straightforward application. The intrinsic value of the sources of organs is contentious, and the instrumental value of organ retrieval strategies is a work in progress.

This is not to say that we cannot evaluate current projects. An overall sound strategy for addressing the problem of premature organ failure must include preventive medicine strategies. Trying to weigh an activity that has been completed is one thing but quite another to weigh something in the midst of a transformation, especially when the transformation itself is difficult to predict. Some people may be inclined to think that, even though we do not know the final results of a project, we can evaluate each project at a given time. Obviously, we can evaluate a project at a given time, but such an evaluation cannot always indicate whether we should abandon or continue that project. If persistent failure indicated that we should abandon a project, transplantation technology would not have become successful.

Struggling through failures and disappointment is a part of progress and what it means to lead a robust human life. In cases of evaluating continuing projects, we are not merely weighing our options and acting on the weightiest option, but committing ourselves to a project with hope, resilience, and creativity. Commitment entails the valuing of a goal even if success is improbable given current conditions and knowledge, a moral stance that is different from merely evaluating the facts, values, and probable success of a project.

9. Conclusion

After scholars address the facts and values of an organ retrieval strategy, we frequently find questionable decisions regarding the prioritization of values. The reason for this is that our current level of moral understanding leaves us in the position where our alternatives are in fact incommensurable. This does not mean that values are incommensurable in principle. Nor does it mean that all of our alternatives are incommensurable. Until moral theorists or applied ethicists set forth a more precise moral methodology, we can expect to find more dubious intuitions, including some of mine, as to what we should do when faced with an ethics case or policy question. I do not foresee anyone developing such a methodology any time soon, and it may not be possible. What we need, then, is an approach to applied ethics that accounts for the uncertainty of outcomes, the incommensurability of values, and the many possibilities available to us in developing a better world.

In summary, we often face incommensurable alternatives resulting from three factors: we have no moral method to prioritize the value of many of our options, we cannot always adequately foresee the consequences of an action or an omission, and we must continually shape the consequences of our actions. Even after we address the facts, values, and probabilities, there will often be great difficulty in prioritizing the values, and in some cases, impossible with our current level of moral understanding. There will often be a gap between the relevant considerations of a case or policy question and the need to determine a unique solution or best response. We must not exaggerate the number of occasions in which we will not be able to determine a best response, but selecting a best course of action will be more difficult than what we generally find in the medical ethics literature. Perhaps the pressure to take a stand on an issue results in authors assuming the commensurability of value.

Constructive pluralism differs from conventional medical ethics in the United States in two significant ways. First, there will be cases where more than one action is permissible because no single action is the best choice. Second, uncertainty and indeterminateness are not merely theoretical remarks but are a feature of real-life cases, practices, and policy decisions. The reason Beauchamp and Childress are right about indeterminateness is that moral decisions are frequently underdetermined by moral reasons. That is, moral reasons justify a moral decision, but it remains debatable whether the reasons are compelling, whether one alternative is the weightiest of feasible options, and to what degree the prospects for attaining a medical goal are realizable. Frequently, moral reasons provide a range of plausible actions but do not indicate which action is morally best.

Part Two

CONFLICTS OF ORGAN RETRIEVAL

Four

TRANSPLANT RECIPIENTS'
QUALITY OF LIFE

As I began studying value conflicts with organ retrieval, I wondered about the diseases causing persons' organs to fail, how those diseases affected those persons' quality of life (QOL), whether organ transplantation improves persons' lives, and about the possibilities of preventing organ failure. Sometimes the causes are unknown, but many diseases leading to organ failure are preventable. Although studies on transplant recipients' quality of life varied in terms of the sample sizes and in their methodologies, the vast majority of commentators agree that organ transplantation significantly improves patients' lives. The information found in this chapter on transplant patients' quality of life represents the literature on transplant recipients' quality of life. All of the medical information in this chapter I borrowed from the Merck Manual unless otherwise indicated.[1] It proved to be an invaluable exposition of technical matters.

To demonstrate the value of organ transplants, transplant patients must have a good opportunity for a quantitatively and qualitatively meaningful post-transplant life. We cannot expect to determine precisely what constitutes a valuable life for transplant patients, but, then, measuring the quality of life for anyone will be imprecise. We can rely on our common sense notion of a valuable life, reports of transplant recipients, and the studies of social scientists. Quality of life studies often have serious shortcomings, but we have sufficient evidence that many transplant recipients lead valuable lives. In this chapter, I present evidence that heart, liver, and kidney transplants are valuable treatments. I do not consider whether the transplantation of other organs is valuable.

First, I briefly address how scholars define and measure transplant patients' quality of life. Second, I note criticisms of quality of life studies. Third, despite these criticisms, anecdotal accounts and social science instruments provide enough evidence that many patients benefit significantly from transplant surgery. I do this by describing the diseases, disorders, and symptoms that lead to transplantation, and the results of transplantation.

No consensus in measuring quality of life or determining what constitutes a good life exists.[2] Most studies attempt to measure quality of life by asking patients to reflect on their physical, psychological, and social well-being. Some explicitly state that we should measure physical functioning in terms of patients' physical symptoms, the frequency of needed medical interventions, and their ability to perform routine tasks.[3] Psychological functioning usually refers to persons' level of well-being, usually indicated by their levels of depression and anxiety.[4] Some of the instruments are general assessments of health and well-being, whereas others address a category of patients such as kidney transplant recipients. One frequently utilized instrument is the Sickness Impact Profile that asks transplant recipients to rate sleep and rest, eating, work, home management, recreation, mobility, ambulation, body care, social interaction, and alertness on a scale from one to five.[5] The summed answers provide a single quality of life score.

Although quality of life instruments convey significant information, studies have serious shortcomings. Despite the many different instruments for measuring quality of life, "Virtually without exception, QOL studies rely exclusively on brief, mailed questionnaires or short interviews; they do not give contextually rich descriptions of the recipients' life circumstances."[6] Some studies make judgments based upon a single questionnaire or post-transplant interview; others summarize data from a series of follow-ups. Many of the studies prejudice the results by waiting a few months after surgery, thereby failing to include those who died miserable deaths after acute rejection. Asking patients to compare their pre-transplant and post-transplant lives can skew the results. Patients' desire to show gratitude to the transplant team inclines them to overestimate their post-transplant well-being.

Despite these shortcomings, we have grounds for concluding that transplants are valuable for many patients. First, the longevity of transplant recipients is objectively measurable. As we will see, the short-term and long-term survival rates for heart, liver, and kidney transplants are impressive. Second, many features of measuring quality of life can be inferred from objective measurements as well such as whether transplant patients work full-time or part-time. Although patients may overestimate their quality of life, we must often believe them when they tell us they feel better after transplantation. This does not mean we should uncritically accept the current data and patient reports, but positive accounts do tell us something positive! The following information indicates the problems besetting transplant patients, while also recognizing the triumphs and reasons for hope.

1. Heart Transplants

Heart transplant candidates usually suffer from cardiomyopathy.[7] Cardiomyopathy progressively impairs the structure or function of the muscular wall of the heart's ventricles. Dilated congestive cardiomyopathy is a group of disorders in which the ventricles enlarge but are unable to pump enough blood for the body. This, in turn, causes heart failure. In the United States, the most common cause of dilated congestive cardiomyopathy is coronary artery disease. Coronary artery disease causes an inadequate blood supply to the heart that impairs the heart. The uninjured part of the heart stretches to compensate for the injury. When this stretching fails to adequately compensate, dilated congestive cardiomyopathy results. Other causes of this disorder include viral infections (most commonly coxsackie virus B), diabetes mellitus, thyroid disease, the abuse of cocaine or antidepressants, and severe and prolonged alcohol abuse.

About 70 percent of patients with dilated congestive cardiomyopathy die within five years of the onset of symptoms that include being short of breath, tiring easily, and chest pain. Treating causes such as alcohol or drug abuse or viral infections can prolong life. Without treatment, the disorder will likely result in death. These facts support the need for heart transplants.

Survival rates for heart transplant recipients at one year are 85 percent; 75 percent at five years; and 70 percent up to ten years.[8] Given this impressive success rate, demonstrating that these patients enjoy a meaningful quality of life proves the value of the procedure, but problems exist.

Transplant patients must take immunosuppressive drugs so that their bodies do not reject the new organ. Long-term use of the immunosuppressive cyclosporine can lead to poisoning of the kidneys, liver, and nervous system, excessive hair growth, osteoporosis, deterioration of veins of the hip, bone fractures, and the growth of tumors. Not surprisingly, patients persistently requested withdrawal of immunosuppressive therapy.[9] Many people have problems with developing a puffy face, acne, tremors, leg cramps, tasting foods, overeating, and sexual dysfunction.[10] Not surprisingly, some patients have experienced deteriorating relationships with spouses and partners after transplantation. Patients may also feel stressed about financial troubles.[11]

Despite possible complications from heart transplantation, an overall evaluation of the procedure and subsequent treatments indicates positive results for many patients. In some studies, heart transplant recipients' quality of life appears too good to be true. One commentator, for example, claims, "Patients report no diminished quality of life as measured by both the Nottingham Health Profile and the General Well-Being examinations."[12] Others make believable-sounding positive claims. Patients experience a higher level of well-being regarding strength and stamina, rest, and sexual intercourse after transplantation. Significant numbers of patients have fewer problems with breathing, heart palpitations, coughing, chest pain, lethargy, fatigue, insomnia, anxiety, depression, and nausea.[13] According to one study, heart transplant recipients achieved as good a functional recovery as patients who underwent coronary artery bypass graft surgery.[14]

Many heart transplant patients have realized dreams and developed meaningful hobbies. Neoral's brochure on heart transplantation mentions several patients who have lived through valuable events: patients have witnessed their children's graduations, gone parasailing, completed graduate degrees, and developed their art work.[15] Presumably, these sorts of events are not restricted to a small minority of heart transplant patients. Doubtless, the brochure is self-interested, but it provides information about the events that constitute a valuable life for transplant patients. Coupled with the aforementioned data on the quality of life of these patients, this shows the value of heart transplantation for many persons.

2. Liver Transplants

Chronic liver disease is the ninth leading cause of death in the United States.[16] Primary biliary cirrhosis, primary sclerosing cholangitis, viral hepatitis, and alcoholic liver disease can all cause liver failure. Others may suffer from familial amyloidotic polyneuropathy, a disease that causes persons to have a sharp decrease in blood pressure when they stand (orthostatic hypotension), gastrointestinal dysfunction, cardiac irregularities and erectile dysfunction.[17] Patients with chronic liver disease suffer from severe fatigue, itching, poor self-esteem, and depression.[18]

Cirrhosis destroys normal liver tissue and leaves nonfunctioning scar tissue. In the United States, the most common cause of cirrhosis is alcohol abuse. Symptoms of cirrhosis include weakness, poor appetite, and weight loss. If bile flow is impeded patients may have jaundice, itching, nodules, a curling up of the fingers, breast enlargement in men, hair loss, abnormal nerve function, and they may vomit blood. Alcoholic cirrhosis is associated with hypertension that enlarges the spleen, fluid accumulation in the abdominal cavity, kidney failure from liver failure, and liver cancer. No cure for cirrhosis exists. Cirrhosis is treatable by withdrawing from alcohol, receiving vitamin supplements, and, in advanced cases, transplantation.

Primary biliary cirrhosis is most common among women between the ages 35 to 60 years, but it can occur in men and women of all ages. The cause of the disease is unknown, but is associated with autoimmune diseases such as rheumatoid arthritis, scleroderma that involves scarring of the skin, joints, and internal organs, blood vessel abnormalities, or inflammation of the thyroid. Primary biliary cirrhosis begins with an inflammation of the bile ducts in the liver that obstructs the flow of bile from the liver. Consequently, the bile remains in the liver or spills into the bloodstream. As the inflammation spreads, so does scar tissue throughout the liver.

Symptoms of primary biliary cirrhosis include fatigue and itching at first. About 50 percent of people with the disease develop an enlarged liver; 25 percent develop an enlarged spleen. A smaller percentage of these patients will have yellow spots in their skin or increased skin pigmentation. Others develop enlarged fingertips and abnormalities of the bone, nerves, and kidneys.

No cure for primary biliary cirrhosis exists, but itching is controllable, and vitamin supplements can help. Patients may need calcium and vitamins A, D, and K because these elements are not well absorbed in cases of insufficient bile. Fortunately, the drug ursodiol apparently slows the progression of the disease. Liver transplantation remains the only option for those in the late stages of the disease.

Primary sclerosing cholangitis causes inflammation and scarring of the liver and obstructs the bile ducts inside and outside the liver. The disease leads to cirrhosis as well. Most persons with this disease are men who have developed inflammatory bowel disease, especially ulcerative colitis, a disease in which the inflammation of the large intestine leads to occurrences of bloody diarrhea, abdominal cramps, and fever. The disease causes fatigue, itching, and jaundice, upper abdominal pain, fluid accumulation in the abdomen, portal hypertension—high blood pressure in the portal vein that brings blood from the intestine to the liver, and liver failure. Afflicted persons may be asymptomatic for up to ten years, but the disease usually worsens. Transplantation offers the best treatment for this fatal disease. In what follows, I present evidence that liver transplantation is valuable.

One study reports the first-year survival rate to be 80 percent and the eight-year survival rate to be 70 percent.[19] Before receiving a liver transplant, patients complain of fatigue, insomnia, and itchy skin. In another study, about half of the patients claimed that one or more of their symptoms was extremely distressing. After transplantation, only a quarter of the patients reported an extremely distressing symptom. Severe pain ratings decreased from 53 to 26 percent. The number of patients who claimed to be very happy increased from 7 percent before transplantation to 42 percent post surgery. To lend perspective to these results, only 33 percent of adults in the general population between the ages 20 and 55 years claimed to be very happy.[20] In a study of transplant recipients treated for familial amyloidotic polyneuropathy, 66 percent were completely satisfied with their liver transplant; 34 percent were partially satisfied.[21] While these are encouraging data, liver transplantation is not without complications.

In one study of 100 transplant recipients, complications included bile leakage, hemorrhaging, hepatic artery thrombosis, kidney failure, and retransplantation for ten patients. Forty-six patients experienced rejection episodes.[22] In another study, liver transplant recipients were twice as likely as members of the general population to report problems with work, housekeeping, social life, hobbies, and vacations.[23] Some claimed their lives were more positive, but others claimed they could not get their hands and feet to work.[24] The same study showed that transplantation improved lives. Many patients reported they were in less pain and that they had fewer functional limits.[25] Although results of liver transplantation are mixed, research suggests that enough patients have survived long enough and well enough for us to conclude that the procedure is often valuable.

3. Kidney Transplants

The one-year transplant survival rate of a living donor kidney is 94.5 percent, and 89 percent for a cadaveric kidney. The five-year kidney transplant survival rate was 78 percent, and 64.7 percent for cadaveric kidneys.[26] Chronic kidney failure may stem from many causes including diabetes, pyelonephritis, hyper-tension-nephrosclerosis, polycystic kidney disease, chronic glomerulonephritis, and arteriosclerosis.[27]

With diabetes mellitus, failure to adequately release or utilize the hormone insulin results in abnormally high levels of blood sugar (glucose). Most diabetes mellitus patients have type II in which the pancreas continues to produce insulin, but the body develops resistance to its effects, causing an insulin deficiency. The disease usually strikes adults over thirty years of age but more frequently ravages the elderly. One risk factor is obesity; 80 to 90 percent of individuals with type II diabetes are obese. Less common causes include high levels of corticosteroids, pregnancy, drugs, and poisons that interfere with the production of insulin. In time, high levels of blood sugar damage blood vessels, nerves, connective tissue, eyes, and kidneys. Diabetes mellitus can cause the kidneys to fail to the point requiring dialysis.

One or both kidneys may have pyelonephritis, a bacterial infection. Infections usually ascend from the urinary tract to the urinary bladder. Infection may spread when kidney stones or an enlarged prostate gland obstructs urine flow thereby preventing the washing out of bacteria. Sometimes the backflow of urine from the bladder into the ureters increases the probability of kidney infection. Other times, the bloodstream carries infections to the kidneys. Symptoms of pyelonephritis include chills, fever, lower back pain, nausea, and vomiting. Chronic pyelonephritis occurs only in people with major abnormalities such as urinary tract obstruction, large persistent kidney stones, or, more commonly, backflow of urine into the ureters in children. This can lead to kidney failure. Physicians usually prescribe antibiotics, or in the case of structural abnormalities, surgery.

Malignant nephrosclerosis is associated with high blood pressure that damages the smallest arteries in the kidneys resulting in kidney failure and damage to the brain or heart. Causes including glomerulonephritis, narrowing of the renal artery, inflammation of kidney blood vessels, and sometimes from hormonal disorders such as pheochromocytoma, Conn's syndrome, or Cushing's syndrome. Symptoms include restlessness, confusion, sleepiness, blurred vision, headache, nausea, and vomiting. Without treatment, about half of the people with malignant nephrosclerosis will die within six months, and most of the others will die within a year. Sixty percent die from kidney failure. Treatment includes lowering blood pressure through diet and drugs. Those with progressive kidney disease are treatable with dialysis.

Polycystic kidney disease is a hereditary disease in which several cysts form in both kidneys causing decreased kidney function. In children, this disease causes the kidneys to enlarge and the abdomen to protrude. Newborns with the disease may die soon after birth because kidney failure prevents the lungs from developing properly. For those who survive, kidney and liver failure eventually occur. In adults, the disease progresses slowly. Symptoms include back pain, blood in the urine, and intense cramping pain from kidney stones. More than 20 percent of these people have dilated blood vessels in the skull. Consequently, 75 percent of these eventually suffer from a brain hemorrhage. More than half of people with this disease develop kidney failure and require dialysis or transplantation. With this in mind, I turn to the quality of life of kidney transplant patients.

In one large study, the results were not favorable. This study examined 520 type I diabetics and 618 non-diabetics. The quality of life scores for nondiabetic transplant recipients were below the fiftieth percentile for the general United States population. For those with diabetes and those who received a kidney-pancreas transplant, the scores were below the twenty-fifth percentile. The diabetic patients reported poor quality of life on physical functioning, general health, and social functioning. Their quality of life was lower than that of persons their age in the general population, but their scores were similar to others with chronic diseases.[28] Other studies paint a better picture.

Kidney transplantation gives patients with end-stage renal disease a better quality of life than those who remain on hemodialysis.[29] Many studies report that kidney transplants improve the quality of life of many patients in many categories.[30] Transplantation enhances quality of life in several ways. First, it frees patients from dialysis. Hemodialysis involves two to three sessions a week and takes from two and a half to five hours each treatment. After transplantation, patients have reported that they have more energy and feel better physically. Patients have few diet restrictions.[31] Some studies have shown that the quality of life improvement is consistent across race and gender.[32] Finally, patients no longer see themselves as chronically ill.[51]

4. Conclusion

Although organ transplantation usually causes mixed results, studies show that many heart, liver, and kidney transplant patients do well long after their surgery. This sufficiently shows the value of the transplantation of hearts, livers, and kidneys. The problem has been that the number of individuals waiting for a transplant exceeds the availability of organs. More than 6,000 persons in the United States died in 2003 while waiting for a transplant. While this number may be fewer than people imagine, all other things remaining equal, we ought to prevent people from dying, especially when they have not had ample opportunity to live a long fulfilling life.

The transplant community has attempted to retrieve or create a sufficient number of organs through several strategies. Some of these practices and proposals are unjustifiable. Even justifiable strategies, though, generate moral losses and residue. These losses provide the basis for new moral reasons and requirements to help these patients while protecting other values. In the next chapter, I focus on routine retrieval, presumed consent, and familial consent in the light of whether we can wrong the dead. The topic highlights problems with making moral decisions when our moral explanations for many persons' deeply held beliefs are suspect.

Five

CAN WE WRONG THE DEAD?

Most of us believe we should treat the dead with respect. We should not defile corpses, we ought to honor wills, and we should keep our promises to people even after they die. At the same time, many people believe that once persons die, no harm can come their way. It should come as no surprise then to learn that practices involving retrieving organs from decedents appear inconsistent. For example, the United States Uniform Anatomical Gift Act (1987) requires the decedent's explicit prior consent or the family's consent to donate, even though failure to gain consent means others will die. In some American states, coroners may legally take corneas as needed unless a family member explicitly objects. Even when the deceased has explicitly expressed a wish to donate through a donor card or driver's license, hospitals permit the family to nullify the donor's former wish. In the light of these apparent discrepancies, I will address two central questions. Can we wrong the dead? Is it wrong to override prior wishes of the dead when considering whether to retrieve their organs?

Many prominent bioethicists believe that either the decedent's prior consent or the family's consent is necessary to justify organ retrieval. Since their treatment is superficial, I address two philosophical positions defending the possibility of wronging the dead that might serve as a premise to defend the moral significance of consent for organ retrieval. First, I analyze the George Pitcher-Joel Feinberg thesis that former persons can be subjects of moral concern.[1] Second, I consider Anthony Serafini's thesis that a former person's properties such as reputations and interests extend beyond a person's life, and these properties warrant moral attention.[2] I argue that the Pitcher-Feinberg thesis and Serafini's thesis are plausible but not convincing. In the end, I consider whether we may justify requiring consent for donation on the basis that it satisfies the preferences of living persons, and that presuming consent or routinely retrieving organs may be wrong on symbolic grounds.

I will use "decedent," "dead person," "dead individual," "the dead," and "corpse" interchangeably. By "presumed consent" I mean the proposal that individuals will have their organs taken unless they explicitly indicate that they do not wish to donate. We can understand "routine retrieval" in a weak sense or a strong sense. The weak sense means that individuals will have their organs taken unless the family objects, but no one attempts to educate persons about an opting out process. Weak routine retrieval is sneaky. The strong sense means that organ retrieval takes place no matter whether the decedent indicated or her family indicates an objection. The term "familial consent" refers to the practice of asking the decedent's family members for permission to retrieve organs.

I am not looking for psychological, sociological, anthropological, or religious reasons that attempt to explain our respect for the dead. The nature of my inquiry is to look for philosophical reasons that justify such respect.

Popular moral theories have difficulty showing why the dead should morally count. Moral standing is usually ascribed to those possessing life, sentience, personhood (entities having some combination of self-awareness, consciousness, and rationality), or the ability to have relationships.[3] Decedents lack these essential properties. They are former persons, not living or future persons.

Consequentialist theories may extend the moral scope to include sentient creatures, but decedents have no actual or potential sentience.[4] Environmental ethics broadens the moral umbrella even further, but usually restricts ethical concern to all living things or necessary parts of biosystems.[5] This move does not cover the dead either.

Any attempt to include non-living things in the moral domain must find some way of limiting the scope of moral concern lest we end up with the absurd view that every speck of dust deserves moral consideration. Another line of thought involves the care that living individuals have for the decedent, but this leaves problems for those no one cares about and assumes rather than proves the value that most of us have placed on dead persons. Despite these initial obstacles, many bioethicists and philosophers defend the view that the dead warrant moral concern.

1. Bioethics and Patient Autonomy

Many bioethicists presume or explicitly argue that respect for the dead can override needs of the living. To justify their position, they appeal to the principle of respect for patient autonomy. Although the value of respecting patients' autonomy is well established, bioethicists fail to explain how this principle applies to cadaveric organ retrieval. Robert Veatch objects to a policy of presumed consent on the basis that it will inevitably violate the former wishes of many dead persons.[6] Since he offers no argument for this premise, it stands as an assumption. Similarly, Arthur Caplan and Beth Virnig claim that presumed consent is more coercive than a policy of presumed non-consent.[7] Even when others argue that presumed consent may be ethically permissible, they often say so on the condition that an effective way to opt-out is necessary.[8]

James Childress says the principle of respect for persons dictates that decedents' former wishes take priority in determining the fate of their organs. The basis for his claim is that wrongdoing does not entail harming, but he omits to explain how we can wrong the dead. Childress then shifts his argument to say that families and religious communities would object to the routine retrieval of persons' organs, but this does not suffice as an adequate reason either, because we can attempt to change their minds or override their objections for the sake of saving lives.[9] Whatever reasons may be stated for thinking justified organ retrieval requires explicit consent, inconsistent practices call for justifiable reasons. And understanding the way we attempt to justify our moral responses is intrinsically valuable.

2. The Pitcher-Feinberg Thesis

Pitcher and Feinberg's arguments defending the view that we can harm dead persons provided the framework for several recent articles. Since Feinberg adopts many of Pitcher's arguments and examples, I will refer to their position as the Pitcher-Feinberg thesis even though they have written separate accounts. This is not to imply that they agree on all points. One difference between Pitcher's and Feinberg's views is that Pitcher uses "harm" to cover instances that are contrary to a desire or interest, while for Feinberg a harm is a special sort of wrong, a setback to an interest.

Pitcher and Feinberg agree on the essentials: the harmed subject's awareness of the harm is not required, and harm to the dead is not a physical process. Since recent commentators most frequently refer to Feinberg's arguments, I will usually refer to Feinberg and utilize his terminology. Because their arguments rest on the same key premises, and they rely on the same examples and intuitions, addressing Feinberg's view also addresses Pitcher's view.

To avoid confusion, Feinberg does not equate harm with being hurt. Again, "harm" is a term of art that means a setback to an interest, while "hurt" means to have a physical pain.[10] He explains that an interest involves an objective good; life and health are examples. Affecting a subject's interests is possible without thwarting or promoting a subject's desires. Feinberg relies on William David Ross's distinction between fulfilling a wish and satisfying a wish.[11] Feinberg clarifies the distinction by saying:

> The fulfillment of a want is simply the coming into existence of that which is desired. The satisfaction of a want is the pleasant experience of contentment or gratification that normally occurs in the mind of the desirer when he believes that his desire has been fulfilled.[12]

He adds that fulfillment does not entail satisfaction: we are often disappointed or left unsatisfied even if our wish comes to fruition. Satisfaction does not entail fulfillment: we can gain satisfaction even if our wish goes unfulfilled in cases where one falsely believes the wish has come to fruition. To his mind, harm occurs based on objective failures of the attainment of wishes instead of the subjective experience of dissatisfaction.[13]

With this in mind, Feinberg adds that another can harm us even if we are unaware of our thwarted desires. He claims, for example, a person can harm his or her spouse by having an adulterous affair, even if the spouse never finds out, because each person has a legal interest in domestic relations and in his or her reputation.[14] This does not help Feinberg's case for how can persons be harmed, if they never find out about their spouse's adulterous affair or about having a bad reputation?

According to Pitcher, persons can be in a state of misfortune by having an incurable fatal disease even if they do not know about it.[15] Here, a person can be harmed without ever finding out about the ailment—a disease can slowly diminish a person's energy, productivity, and happiness without the person ever realizing it. Since Pitcher and Feinberg believe living persons can experience harm without being aware of the harm, they do not find it counter intuitive to claim that we can harm the dead when their former wishes are thwarted.[16] *Prima facie*, their examples do not address the problem that while living persons can be adversely affected by circumstances unknown to them, dead persons cannot be physically affected at all. How can individuals be harmed if they cannot be physically or psychologically affected? What interests do they have that can be set back?

Both Pitcher and Feinberg recognize the need to explain how a present or future event can harm a dead individual. Neither Pitcher nor Feinberg wants to ground his argument on the possibility of a retroactive harm because it suggests retroactive causation, causes that move backward in time.[17] They circumvent the problem of retroactive causation by claiming posthumous harms do not involve causation at all.[18] To establish this point, Pitcher offers, and Feinberg adopts, the distinction between an ante-mortem person after his death and a post-mortem person after his death. In Pitcher's words:

> Consider the linguistic act of describing a dead person. There are two different things a person might do if he sets out to describe a friend of his who is now dead: (a) he can describe the dead friend as he was at some stage of his life—i.e., as a living person. (b) he can describe the dead friend as he is now, in death—mouldering, perhaps, in a grave. In (a), we may say that there is a description of an *ante*-mortem person after his death, while in (b) there is a description of a *post*-mortem person after his death. I maintain that although both ante-mortem and post-mortem persons can be described after their death, only ante-mortem persons can be wronged after their death.[19]

The post-mortem person is the person who has been cremated or whose corpse is about to be, as Pitcher puts it, so much dust. No one can harm a post-mortem person. The ante-mortem person is the person who was once alive whom Pitcher and Feinberg believe we can harm or wrong. Although

Pitcher does not address the issue of respect for decedents' prior wishes to donate their organs, he explicitly claims ante-mortem persons can be wronged, for instance, if while alive they were promised to be buried in their respective family plots, but were actually sold to a medical school for dissection.[20] Presumably, Pitcher would think the same conclusion holds true in cases where individuals do not want their organs taken after death but have their ante-mortem wishes violated through a policy of presumed consent or a case where people knowingly transgress the decedent's previous wishes. His point also appears to apply in cases where families do not consent to a decedent's prior wish to donate. I do not know whether Feinberg would agree with this example, but he does agree with Pitcher's general philosophical point.

To support the possibility of harming ante-mortem persons, Pitcher and Feinberg explain that individuals can be, and often are, in a harmed condition before the actualization of the harm.[21] This may appear counterintuitive, but Pitcher offers some interesting analogies. One analogy, which I have updated, is that if some catastrophic event destroys the world during the United States presidency immediately after George Walker Bush, it will be true then and now that George W. Bush is the penultimate president of the United States.[22]

Similarly, Feinberg says that if all of a person's investments should irreparably collapse after his death, it harms his present interest in contributing to the welfare of his loved ones.[23] The underlying point is significant and worth making explicit. A claim about a present state of affairs can become true by a future event even though the future event remains unknown and was not predicted. The second example also suggests the possibility of harming a person who does not suffer from any adverse consequences.

Despite Pitcher's and Feinberg's ornate argumentation and interesting examples, their argument stands deficient. Both Pitcher and Feinberg rely heavily on analogies and hypothetical cases to elicit intuitions that we can wrong dead persons. Their analogies show that preference satisfaction and subjective awareness are not necessary for harm when we construe harm as a setback to an interest. They have shown that harm does not always involve causal relations. What these analogies show is that some initial obstacles to thinking we can harm the dead depend on conditions thought to be necessary for harm, and yet reflection demonstrates these conditions are not necessary.

One problem is that Pitcher and Feinberg rely heavily on intuitive cases about posthumous harms. The idea is to show that the preponderance of the moral evidence indicates we can harm the dead. Perhaps they believe that once we overcome the apparent obstacles to believing in posthumous harms, intuitions about cases provide all the needed moral evidence. The limitation with this strategy is that it leaves open the possibility that other thoughtful individuals may not share their intuitions. If we have learned anything about epistemology this century, intuitions cannot serve as an unshakeable foundation for beliefs because justification takes place within a body of belief. At a less theoretical level, our intuitions may be nothing more than prejudices. In contrast to Pitcher and Feinberg who offer examples and cases to elicit intuitions that we can harm or wrong the dead, Joan Callahan attempts to bring forth counter intuitions.

3. Callahan's Challenge

According to Callahan, "If we feel at all sorry for the dead in such cases, it is not because we think that while alive the person was harmed—indeed, it is common to express relief that the living (ante-mortem) person was not harmed by whatever the event is."[24] Callahan acknowledges our tendency to think we can wrong the dead, but she does not think this is a genuine moral intuition. In emotivist fashion, she explains that our beliefs that we can violate the dead are strictly emotional responses, There can be no philosophical reason for thinking we can harm the dead. She believes we are misled because the value of respecting the wishes of the dead usually cohere with other valuable events such as securing the well-being of heirs, and comforting family members. She notes that we would not be willing to carry out the wishes of artists, presumably talented ones, who wanted their work burned after their death, or honor the wishes of those who wanted others to euthanize the dead person's healthy dog.[25] Regarding the possibility of damaging a dead person's reputation, say, Albert Einstein, Callahan believes Einstein's reputation for genius is not a characteristic of the ante-mortem or post-mortem Einstein. Instead, the reputation is a trait of those appraising Einstein's scientific work.

Callahan considers whether we should attempt to alter our sentiments regarding the treatment of the dead and whether we should change American laws accordingly. She concludes that we should not change the laws because current widespread beliefs and practices comfort the living.[26] But given the shortage of organs available for transplantation, we can make a case that our sentiments and laws should change for the sake of transplant candidates.

Would Callahan have us respect the wishes of dead talented artists who wanted their artwork buried with them? If so, how would she make that cohere with her claim that we should refuse to burn the work? If not, why should we allow persons to take their organs to the grave? While Callahan's arguments advance the debate, Serafini raises significant challenges.

4. Serafini's Thesis

Serafini thinks Callahan's example of the artists and the dog owners are misleading. Defenders of the view that we should honor decedents' prior wishes need not commit themselves to the view that we should always respect their former wishes. Other values can override or cancel the former wishes of the dead. Defenders of the view that the dead can be wronged only need to believe that, all other things being equal, the dead should have their former wishes honored. The value of appreciating art and the value of the dog's life override or cancel the decedents' prior wishes. Callahan's examples only show that we should not honor some wishes of the dead; they do not show the impossibility of wronging the dead. To this extent, I agree with Serafini.

Serafini also believes Callahan goes wrong in thinking that harm must be committed against a whole person. He instructs us to shift our attention away from the decedent to properties the decedent once possessed that continue beyond the person's life. Although Serafini recognizes the temptation to presume an "entity must exist contemporaneously with its properties," he adduces several reasons for thinking otherwise. Serafini prefers "properties" to Feinberg's "interests" because properties, and not interests, are what make things what they are.[27] In this way, Serafini thinks he can circumvent Callahan's criticism that the Pitcher-Feinberg thesis resurrects strange ontological entities, namely, ante-mortem and post-mortem selves.

Only living entities have interests, but all things—including dead persons—have properties. Serafini believes a person's properties live on not merely in the memories of those still living but as things that can be the subject of moral concern. Such properties linger, he thinks, the way a coffee's aroma does after the cup is empty, or the way after-images persist when the TV has been turned off, or the way a black hole still has a gravitational pull although the star has ceased to exist.[28] Similarly, a person's reputation lives on even after he or she dies, or so Serafini believes.

To bolster his argument, Serafini claims that the view that we can wrong the dead coheres with broader beliefs about language. He challenges Callahan's argument that posthumous reputations are appraisals made by living persons about the decedent's previous life. Serafini says such a move implies that living persons do not have reputations either.[29] He expects us to reject this apparent consequence, but we could bite the bullet and say living persons do not have reputations. Instead, talk about reputations is merely an economical way of commenting on how individuals perceive and judge others. Alternatively, we could attempt to show that while living persons have reputations, dead people do not. In what follows, I explore these two strategies.

Serafini believes recasting claims about a person's reputation in terms of how others regard them is to introduce an *ad hoc* hypothesis; a hypothesis that lacks evidence and is summoned only to salvage the belief. For the case at hand, opponents of the view that we can wrong the dead introduce the hypothesis that we should understand persons' reputations solely in terms of appraisers' beliefs only to support the idea that we cannot wrong the dead. But unless we have good reasons for believing we should understand persons' reputations this way, independent of the belief that we cannot wrong the dead, the move is fallacious.

One attempt to avoid the *ad hoc* fallacy would be to see if such a belief squares with other linguistic intuitions. Serafini believes looking to broader linguistic usage suggests otherwise. For example, he claims that saying "bigamy is moral" attempts to describe bigamy even if it can also be said to mean that some community of evaluators believes that bigamy is moral. The two positions are not mutually exclusive. Similarly, he believes when someone claims that a decedent's reputation has been damaged, the claim is about what the living believe about the dead person's reputation. Serafini believes that although some properties that living persons have such as intelligence and kindness cease when a person dies, death does not extinguish all morally relevant properties.[30]

Serafini's argument is interesting and worth clarifying. If we can establish that dead persons have reputations, then dead persons can have damaged reputations. If we can wrongly damage reputations, we can wrongly damage the possessor of the reputation. The linguistic evidence suggests that dead persons have reputations and we can wrong them. If we can wrong dead persons, then we will be in good position to argue that we can wrong dead persons when we ignore their prior wishes regarding organ donation.

The weak link in Serafini's argument is his claim that linguistic intuitions support the notion that dead persons have reputations. He supports the notion by looking to linguistic analogies. The challenge is to find claims sufficiently similar to claims about damaged reputations so that his analogies are appropriate. This will not be easy—what claims are sufficiently similar to claims about damaging a dead person's reputation? Serafini believes some moral claims suffice. He does not believe that we can construe all moral claims as strictly psychological claims about the appraisers. I agree. We must wonder, though, whether claims about harming posthumous reputations are sufficiently similar to Serafini's example about bigamy.

We do not have to revive logical positivism to realize that taking subject-predicate relations too seriously can lead to unnecessary metaphysical puzzles. Bad linguistic habits mean that we do not always say what we mean or mean what we say. Because some speech habits become socially entrenched does not make them good tools to settle metaphysical or moral disputes. We may coherently think that if a person never becomes aware of having a negative reputation, and no adverse consequences to that person result, it precludes harm to the person. So why should we prefer Serafini's linguistic intuitions?

Consider whether saying dead persons do not have reputations implies that living persons lack them as well. Suppose, for example, someone says, "the professor has skeptical students." To my mind, this statement economically expresses that skeptical students have registered for a class taught by the professor. With this rendition, we do not have to claim that having skeptical students is one of the professor's properties. Some persons may insist the speaker is attributing the property of being the teacher of skeptical students to the professor; that this is a property of the professor. Even if this move holds water, we can push the point as it relates to the possibility of wronging the dead.

Suppose that after the professor dies, someone at the funeral says, "as the minister prayed, the dead professor's skeptical students listened with one eye open." It violates good sense to think that the deceased professor has skeptical students; the apostrophe does not fool us. Given the opportunity to introduce themselves, they could say they were the deceased's students, not that they are the deceased's students. Even if they introduce themselves as the professor's students, we can construe their remarks as meaning that they were once the professor's students.

Even if we believe reputations are the sorts of things that individuals possess, I do not see any reason to think dead persons possess them. Serafini may not be correct in believing that denying dead persons have reputations implies living persons do not possess them either. Neither does such a view appear *ad hoc* in the light of some of our linguistic beliefs since several properties obviously cease when the subject dies. At best, the linguistic evidence for posthumous reputations appears inconclusive. It may not be that we can wrong the dead by damaging their reputations. Commentators have still not proven that we can wrong the dead.

5. Symbolic Action and the Preferences of the Living

Among those writing about organ retrieval or organ transplantation, William May offers an interesting and spirited defense of the view that we have reasons to respect the dead.[31] May emphasizes the connection between human dignity and our ability to feel horror when confronted with a dead body. The inability to shudder at the mutilation of the dead is not a healthy rational response, but a mark of inhumanity. Similarly, routinely retrieving organs may suppress or blunt our ability for appreciating the horror of death. Since the horror of death and the belief that the dead can be mistreated remain deep within many persons' psyche, they cannot readily change their attitudes to accommodate routine retrieval. May likens routine retrieval to devouring the corpse—a symbolic message bound to erode the trust in hospitals as centers of healing. Routinely taking organs also violates the continuity between the deceased and his or her family. In May's eloquent words:

> The funeral service (which includes fitting disposition of the corpse) presupposes and reinforces a certain continuity between the person, his mortal remains, and the family unit. This continuity is particularly prominent while the newly dead body has its recognizable form; it attenuates when the body returns to particles. Thus funeral rites are an expression of the continuity of the soul with its body and with the gathered community of friends, colleagues, and family . . . . The corpse, the de-

ceased, and the family belong, as it were, to a continuum which should enjoy a certain sanctuary against the larger society and the state.[32]

May repeatedly speaks about coercively taking organs against families' wishes and of the symbolic value of the proper disposal of the dead. We can agree with May that we should be sensitive to the decedent's living family members. We can also agree that the person's passage from life to death and our treatment of the dead body has powerful symbolic value. But May's observations raise more interesting questions than they answer.

Why cannot we change our attitudes about routine retrieval and presumed consent when organ transplantation realizes a significant social good? Why should we think that presumed consent or routine retrieval would erode faith in hospitals as centers of healing when they would take organs to save lives and when regulations prevent transplant team members from making healthcare decisions for potential donors? What is the moral import of symbolic actions when actions can have multiple meanings and conflicting interpretations?

Perhaps surprisingly, Feinberg argues that we can change our attitudes regarding the treatment of the dead for the sake of increasing the supply of available organs for transplantation. He believes our reluctance to accept presumed consent and routine retrieval is due to our aesthetic sensibilities. I take it that he means we feel something disrespectful and, perhaps, disgusting about retrieving organs from dead persons without their prior consent, even for the purpose of saving lives. Feinberg couches the distaste that many have for these proposals in terms of sentimental attachment to the symbolic value of the human body. He believes much of the current aesthetic aversion is similar to when earlier generations protested against autopsies for resolving crimes or for protecting the public's health, and when writers of the nineteenth century called abdominal surgeons inhuman.[33]

Feinberg sympathizes with May's point that our sense of human dignity remains intimately connected with our ability to experience horror. He says, "to be sure persons sometimes need to 'learn how to shudder,' but it is even more commonly the case that people have to learn how not to shudder."[34]

According to Feinberg, we should be much more concerned with obtaining the needed organs than we are with violating aesthetic sensibilities regarding treatment of the dead. He says organ removal is no worse a fate for a human body than rotting in the ground or burning by flames.[35] Although he mentions autopsies, he could have added that autopsies involve more invasive procedures than organ retrieval. Since we approve of autopsies and many of us will have our bodies autopsied, we cannot rationally object to becoming organ donors on the basis that it involves a grotesque process. Aesthetic affronts only partially explain some people's objection to becoming donors.

I suspect that organ donation violates many persons' sense of individuality, a sense reinforced by the transplant recipient's natural reaction to reject the new organ. Many of us want a sense of wholeness—a unified self at some level. Organs are not only functional parts but symbolic of us as a complete person, and, for whatever reasons, we want to keep that sense of wholeness in life and death. Perhaps we retain a belief that fragmented selves cannot properly "rest" in death if their organs live on in others. These considerations show that the moral significance of organ retrieval includes concerns about the symbolic value of giving and taking organs. Still, this does not show that presumed consent and routine retrieval are morally impermissible, especially when we accept autopsies as morally permissible.

Given the value of extending life, why do we not take organs as we need them regardless of dead persons' prior wishes? All fifty American states allow coroners to remove corneas from the dead without the decedent's or the family's consent.[36] Why corneas, but not hearts and livers? Is it merely because taking corneas is easier to keep clandestine? Why do we allow families to override the decedent's wish to donate when the Uniform Anatomical Gift Act makes transplantation permissible when the deceased has given prior consent?

Apparently, healthcare providers worry about legal liability, fear undermining public support for organ transplantation, and wish to respect the surviving family.[37] I see no reason for thinking the removal of decedents' organs against their prior wishes is any worse than choosing not to utilize persons' healthy organs when they have consented. Given that taking organs saves lives, failing to retrieve organs when the newly dead have previously consented is morally worse than overriding a decedent's wish not to donate.

6. For the Living

Perhaps the only moral basis for respecting the wishes of the dead is for the sake of the living. On this account, seeking consent of the decedent's family would make more sense. Even if we respect the dead for the sake of the living, no obvious reason to seek the family's consent exists. We might argue, for example, that public opinion should have the final say. It would be puzzling if most people would tolerate or accept routine retrieval, and not become donors in an altruistic system, but maybe they would.

Alternatively, utilitarian calculations may suggest, after all, that if most living individuals believe we should retrieve organs as needed, we should carry it out. Still, it may be argued that we have a deontological reason to retrieve organs even without the decedent's prior consent or family's consent for the sake of extending life for those in need. We would have to think of the social consequences of such policies. I would not want us to dismiss families' wishes, but justifying our practice of familial consent appears difficult—it serves neither respect for the dead nor the greatest public good. Though May speaks of the symbolic power of giving the deceased over to their families, organ retrieval from those who agree to donation neither disrupts American funeral rituals nor conveys disturbing messages about our insensitivity toward the dead or the illegitimate use of state power. We must question why routine retrieval or presumed consent is more objectionable than routine autopsies when people die under suspicious circumstances.

Interestingly, presumed consent and routine retrieval convey disturbing messages for some. Recall May's comment that routine retrieval is like devouring the corpse. I guess for May and others such policies utilize people like meat for the sake of others. In contrast, autopsies serve a significant social good and the interests of the dead person's family. Family members of murder victims, for instance, want the murderer or murderers brought to justice. Many persons have the mystical belief that victims will "rest" better knowing that the killer or killers have been captured, prosecuted, and sentenced. Still, we can question whether the symbolic value of respecting the dead overrides the needs of transplant candidates and their families. After all, transplantation serves a significant social good as well.

One might say that the burden of proof rests on those who advocate routine retrieval, presumed consent, or familial consent. After all, those who defend routine retrieval or presumed consent are the ones bucking tradition. Tradition, although not sacrosanct, carries moral weight, because habits create comfort and expectations. Changes may result in the deterioration of happiness and undermine what sense of community remains, thereby exacerbating much of the alienation experienced in modern societies. Conversely, we should try to better understand our practices, and understanding is not possible without genuine criticism. Although tradition carries moral weight, so do new possibilities brought about by new technologies that call us to reevaluate our beliefs, values, and practices.

7. Conclusion

Contemporary attempts to show we can wrong the dead have not been successful, but I have not abandoned my belief that we have a moral requirement to treat the dead with respect. The problem with justifying respect for the dead stems from narrow moral theories. The problem with justifying respect for dead organ donors stems from the questionable attempt to rely on the model of respect for patient autonomy. For several reasons, these difficulties do not mean we should rush to change laws or policies to embrace routine retrieval or presumed consent.

First, our intuition that we can wrong the dead can be true even if we lack compelling arguments and explanations. Second, if we decide to ignore the prior wishes of the dead and take their organs anyway as in the case of corneas, then many of the living will suffer emotionally. We have only to witness grieving family members when they find out that the coroner took their loved one's corneas without their or the decedent's consent. Third, routine re-

trieval and presumed consent might instigate a backlash against the organ retrieval community. Fourth, we can manipulate the availability of transplantable organs in many ways: by redefining death, selling organs, developing
xenotransplants and stem cell research. Until we consider all of these strategies, we will not know whether routine retrieval or presumed consent is necessary or a good option. The practice of gaining familial consent when the decedent has indicated the wish to donate is unjustifiable.

Ultimately, I hope that consideration of the moral status of the dead will
encourage us to think more broadly about what it means to have moral standing and what implications this has for medical ethics. This chapter also raised
interesting issues as to whether we are willing and able to make necessary legal, social, and psychological adjustments to accommodate routine retrieval,
presumed consent, and to abandon familial consent. In the subsequent chapters, I discuss other major organ retrieval strategies that highlight my emphasis on many possible adjustments to the problem of premature or congenital
organ failure. In the next chapter, I further demonstrate this moral complexity
by discussing the definition of death.

Six

DEFINING DEATH

Prior to the 1950s, the permanent cessation of a person's heart and lungs constituted necessary and sufficient conditions for death. In the late 1960s, the meaning of death changed from a cardiopulmonary definition to a brain definition because respirators can indefinitely maintain heart and lung function. Those who accept a brain definition have divided into two camps. Whole brain advocates, as the words suggest, believe all significant brain processes must cease for persons to die. Their challenge is to distinguish significant from insignificant brain processes without sounding arbitrary. Conversely, higher brain defenders argue that the loss of brain functions that lead to the end of the individual human being qua human being constitute death—this is equated with the permanent loss of consciousness or personal identity. The apparent problems are that we do not require consciousness in other organisms to determine them alive, and we must then regard permanently unconscious persons whose vegetative functions persist as dead. An individual could also undergo a complete personality change without dying. The loss of personal identity is not sufficient for death.

There has also been considerable discussion as to whether artificial life support brought about a new definition of death or merely a new criterion for determining death.[1] This literature tends to be more confusing than helpful because authors simplify distinctions between empirical and conceptual issues. I use "definition of death" instead of "criterion for death," because commentators use "definition" more frequently in the literature, and I assume that a change in use signifies a change in meaning.

The debate over the cardiopulmonary, the whole brain, and the higher brain definitions of death spawned several intriguing and difficult questions. Given the difficulties scientists and physicians have had with defining death with precision, should we look outside science for answers? Is defining death a moral issue? How do we know precisely when organ retrieval is permissible? Answers remain elusive after thirty years of debate.

1. Historical Background for the Whole Brain Definition of Death

During the 1950s, the world faced a poliomyelitis epidemic that killed many children by restricting their ability to breathe. Physicians utilized air bags to pump oxygen into children's lungs, a process at first performed manually. Later, respirators or ventilators better performed this task, proving beneficial for other patients as well, including accident victims who remained comatose.[2] As a consequence of artificial ventilation, healthcare providers could indefinitely continue heart and lung functioning in persons who otherwise appeared lifeless. Withdrawing life support from these unfortunate patients led people to reconsider the nature of death.

Performing heart transplants also stimulated a reexamination of death. The retrieval of the heart must take place as soon as possible after the donor dies to preserve the organ. People realized vegetative patients whose heart and lung functioning was being mechanically maintained could provide a good source of organs, but withdrawing treatment had to be morally justified.[3]

Unless the definition of death changed, taking organs from vegetative patients would be murder, since cardiopulmonary functioning, even though mechanically maintained, meant that the patient had not yet died by the heart-lung definition. For these reasons, the medical community doubted the heart-lung definition and looked for an alternative.

The cardiopulmonary definition lost ground as attention shifted to the brain. In the United States, the impetus for a transition to a brain definition came in 1968 from the Ad Hoc Committee of the Harvard Medical School. The committee proposed several medical tests to establish death. First, the subject should be completely unaware of stimuli. Unresponsiveness to painful stimuli will lend strong support that this condition has been satisfied. Second, doctors should observe that the subject has no spontaneous muscular movement or respiration for one hour. Third, the subject's eyes should remain dilated; blinking should be absent. Fourth, there should be no evidence of swallowing, yawning, or vocalization. Fifth, the subject should exhibit a flat electroencephalogram (EEG). They recommended the repetition of these tests twenty-four hours later, and physicians should be able to rule out alternative diagnoses such as hypothermia or damage resulting from nervous system depressants. If the subject meets these conditions, physicians should declare death and terminate artificial respiration. They should then observe the individual for three minutes after terminating the respirator.[4]

This shift meant accepting a conception of death in which the brain no longer functioned, other organs remained viable, and withdrawing treatment could be justified. In this way, physicians could avoid prosecution for terminating medical treatment for a living patient.[5] Shortly thereafter, the brain death definition was widely accepted in the United States.

The shift from a cardiopulmonary definition to a brain definition made sense at the time. As the President's Commission of 1981 pointed out, "the brain cannot regenerate neural cells to replace ones that have permanently stopped metabolizing."[6] The technology of the day could not mimic brain functioning.

Since the cardiopulmonary view no longer appeared sound, some plausible alternative had to take its place. As the regulator of organic activity in higher organisms, the brain became the focal point in understanding death.

Given the complexity of the brain, though, the medical community needed a better grasp of what constitutes brain death.

Brain death means the death of the whole brain. Traditional wisdom divided the brain into higher and lower functions. The higher brain was associated with the cerebrum since it primarily controls consciousness, thought, memory, and feeling; the lower brain with the brain stem as it controls lower functions such as swallowing, yawning, sleep-wake cycles, and respiration. The distinction helps clarify why the destruction of the brain stem constitutes whole brain death. The destruction of the brain stem deprives the heart of oxygen, and the signs of life will cease without artificial support.[7]

The Commission cautioned that the higher-lower distinction oversimplifies complex interactions within the brain. According to the President's Commission, the medical community entertained two views of whole brain death. The first view looks at the heart, lungs, and brain as significant for life because the cessation of any of these organs begins the demise of the organism's integrated functioning.[8] Supposedly, the brain takes primacy in this configuration, but the Commission did not clarify why.

The second view gives full prominence to the brain on the basis that it regulates the functioning of the entire organism. This view implies that when a brain-dead subject receives artificial support, breathing and circulation continue as mere artifacts instead of an indicator of integrated functioning. Although the Commission believed that the two views differed only in degree, they believed the first formulation to be preferable for practical purposes.[9] They thought that emphasizing the brain's integrative functioning satisfied medical experts' view equating brain death with death and lay persons' view that death entails the cessation of cardiopulmonary functioning.[10] Consequently, the definition accepted by the commission reads as follows:

> An individual is dead who has sustained either irreversible cessation of circulatory and respiratory functions, or irreversible cessation of all functions of the entire brain, including the brain stem.[11]

They also made explicit that a determination of death must accord with accepted medical standards.

Other influential groups including the American Bar Association, the American Medical Association, and the National Conference of Commissioners on Uniform State Laws have also endorsed the brain death definition.[12]

2. Problems with the Whole Brain Definition of Death

In the United States, neurosurgeons and neurologists do not always agree on brain death criteria. In one study, even sixteen years after the acceptance of brain death, neurosurgeons and neurologists utilized different criteria to declare death: 88 percent required the absence of pupillary reflex and 61 percent required an absence of the cough reflex. Nor does the American public understand brain death well. People frequently confuse brain death with coma or persistent vegetative state or believe that cardiac function must cease before declaring death.[13] Experts on brain death disagree on the acceptability of whole brain death as well.

Critics of the whole brain definition point out that the entire brain does not cease when a person is dead under whole brain standards. Robert Truog points out that many persons diagnosed as brain dead still exhibit electrical activity on their EEGs.[14] Consequently, whole brain defenders must decide which brain activities and functions are significant to determine whether a person has died. Robert Veatch plausibly argues that they must draw some arbitrary lines between brain stem and spinal cord activity, and, within the brain, decide whether cellular activity constitutes functioning.[15]

More significant for present purposes, Truog states, "clinicians have observed that patients who fulfill the tests for brain death frequently respond to surgical incision at the time of organ procurement with a significant rise in both heart rate and blood pressure."[16] This observation sounds as if surgeons are retrieving organs from living, albeit severely compromised, persons. We could interpret this observation as dead persons having physiological responses just as we note that the dead still develop goose bumps when cold. These apparent anomalies motivate some to seek an alternative definition of death.

3. The Higher Brain Definition

Higher brain defenders disagree with the way whole brain advocates frame the issue. Richard Zaner thinks that whole brain advocates avoid asking, who died?[17] One camp within the higher brain school believes this question must account for individuals' psychological traits. Hugo Tristram Engelhardt, for example, says that if we think that in living a life where we breathe, but not much else, and we believe that such a life is not worth living and that we would not be present, then we have taken a major step toward the higher brain position.[18] These higher brain defenders believe the permanent loss of a person's identity constitutes death.

If, in the future, all body parts including the entire brain were transplantable, then individuals who receive an entirely new body with accompanying new psychological and physical properties would no longer be the same persons. The former persons as unique blends of psychological and physical traits with their histories are dead, but the new persons are assuredly not dead. The permanent cessation of personal identity is not sufficient for the death of a psychological-physical-historical organism. When we ask whether an individual is dead, we refer to a complex set of interactions of mind, body, and history. For this reason, regarding death as the permanent cessation of an individual's personal identity is fraught with conceptual problems that will invariably lead to practical problems.

Other higher brain advocates make personhood instead of personal identity necessary and sufficient for human life. That is, the qualities that make an individual a person worthy of moral respect are necessary and sufficient for that individual being alive. Since consciousness and cognition are required for personhood, and such abilities are associated with the cerebral hemispheres—especially the neocortex—some scholars equate death with the destruction of the neocortex. Veatch has pointed out that in principle a microcomputer could replace the neocortex as the cause of consciousness. Veatch believes a person dies if and only if the person loses consciousness forever.[19]

The higher brain position contradicts many persons' view that other organisms need not be conscious to be alive. I do not find the higher brain definition convincing. It appears to me that we lack compelling reason to think death means different things for different organisms. I regard death as a biological event and persistently vegetative patients as alive. Our common sense view of death entails that the body ceases—largely—along with the mind. Determining the extent is the hard part, and further inquiry might not resolve the debate. Given the difficulties with the whole brain and higher brain definitions, some recommend a return to the cardiopulmonary definition or attempt to rehabilitate the whole brain definition.

4. Revisiting the Whole Brain Definition

James Bernat has developed a more sophisticated version of the whole brain definition. Again, the whole brain definition runs into difficulties because those who satisfy whole brain death still exhibit apparent signs of life. To summarize, these include electrical activity detectable by an EEG, the production of hormones, and a rise in blood pressure during organ retrieval. Bernat attempts to offer a whole brain position that overcomes this apparent counter-evidence.

Bernat says we must first agree on the meaning of death. In his words, physicians cannot determine whether a person is dead "until first there is agreement on the meaning of death in a new technological world where continuation of designated lost vital functions can be performed artificially."[20] Bernat concedes that not all brain functions cease when a person dies, so he defines death as "the permanent cessation of the critical functions of the organism as a whole."[21] In turn, he uses "critical function" in reference to "the extent to which a given function of the organism as a whole is necessary for the maintenance of life, health, and unity of the organism."[22] For Bernat, three functions are critical: spontaneous breathing and autonomic control of circulation, homeostasis, including appropriate responses to baroreceptors, chemoreceptors, neuroendocrine feedback loops, and similar systems, and consciousness required for hydration, nutrition, and protection.[23]

The reason for the second critical function is that baroreceptors detect and communicate blood pressure; chemoreceptors recognize the presence of chemical compounds; and neuroendocrine feedback loops regulate hormones. Destruction of the whole brain (both hemispheres, diencephalon, and the brain stem) satisfies these conditions. The brain stem controls respiration and circulation, the brain stem and hypothalamus control the critical functions, and the cerebral cortex, thalamus, and brain stem control consciousness.[24] Based on these criteria, the production of antidiuretic hormone does not count as a critical function because "patients without such secretion can survive for long periods without treatment."[25]

Although Bernat makes an ambitious and plausible case, we must consider reasons for thinking he has not settled the debate. Bernat's third critical function—consciousness related to nutrition, hydration, and protection—is difficult to understand. Consciousness is not necessary for biological life, and Bernat regards death as strictly a biological phenomenon. It would have made more sense for Bernat to say, "brain function related to nutrition, hydration, and protection is critical."

Nor do I believe, as Bernat does, that once we have a good definition of death we can always establish whether a human being is dead, even if the tests we utilize are valid.

Twentieth-century philosophy of science has sufficiently established to my mind the impossibility of neatly demarcating empirical statements from definitions. I will not revisit these arguments, but the implication is that we cannot establish necessary and sufficient conditions for terms such as "death" independently from a broader web of considerations that include an appraisal of words' meanings and of the empirical evidence. In this case, we cannot establish the meaning of death apart from our views about which persons are dead. Criteria and tests for establishing death remain in reflective equilibrium with our intuitions regarding which people are dead in a variety of contexts. Stuart J. Younger, for example, tells of patients who satisfy criteria for whole brain death except for the apnea test because they spontaneously breathe periodically.[26] To Younger and me, these people are dead. Bernat's list of critical functions does not cover all cases.

New neurophysiological findings have further complicated the debate. Just as the medical community has developed ways to induce heart-lung functioning in brain-injured persons indefinitely, they have also found ways to artificially mimic brain function. In a 1986 article, Japanese doctors reported that brain dead people lack a hormone that constricts blood vessels. Doctors found that when they fed this hormone to brain dead individuals, they sustained them for an average of twenty-three days.[27] Some brain functions are amenable to artificial control just as the respirator mimics the heart and lungs. Technological developments cast serious doubt on the way we determine and define death. The difficulties with precisely determining death in all contexts have led some bioethicists to think that defining and declaring death is not merely a scientific-medical issue.

5. Is Defining Death a Moral Issue?

Karen Gervais and Veatch have each abandoned the idea of finding a single or cluster of anatomical facts to settle the dispute over defining death. Gervais and Veatch claim that the debate is a moral issue. They suggest we add a conscience clause to the officially accepted definition so that individuals and their families can choose a definition consistent with their values and views.[28]

In the United States, New Jersey and New York, for example, allow persons to reject the whole brain definition on religious grounds.[29] I am inclined to disagree with Gervais and Veatch, but I do believe that they raise interesting issues relevant to my discussion of value conflicts, moral losses, and residue. Over the years, Veatch has advanced three arguments to support the point, but I will focus on his suggestion that choosing a definition of death entails significant moral consequences.[30]

One assumption that leads Veatch to view the definition of death as a moral issue is that he believes the issue has become a line-drawing problem. Veatch correctly notes that technology has greatly extended the temporal length between indicators of death such as loss of breath and blood flow and the death of the brain.[31] We face the difficulty of deciding where along this extended time line conditions sufficiently and necessarily indicate death.

Veatch believes that appropriately pronouncing death requires temporal precision because significant consequences flow from declaring death. Since technological advances in making precise body function measurements has shown that organs do not all cease simultaneously, he believes no single physiological event can precisely define the moment of death for all cases. He proposes we define death as the moment when a cluster of death behaviors becomes appropriately set in motion.[32] We cannot always exactly determine the *facticity* of the timing of death, but we must still decide what we *ought* to do with persons at each stage of their fuzzy existence between life and death.

Different definitions fix the time of death differently resulting in different implications for when familial and community death behaviors ought to be set in motion. At times, though, scholars have exaggerated the moral significance of defining death. Consider the double-edged worries of Veatch, for example. On the one hand, Veatch worries that if we declare someone dead there will be no more treatment alternatives. He does not want treatment terminated against persons' prior wishes or their family's wishes based upon a debatable definition of death.[33] Conversely, he cautions against drawing the line too late because that would waste medical resources on hopeless individuals and lose the opportunity to transplant organs.[34]

Amir Halevy and Baruch Brody express a similar concern, but they rightly argue that we can separate both in concept and in practice withdrawing and withholding treatment from defining death.[35] We do not want to treat dead bodies. We also have many good reasons to terminate futile treatment. So we do not need to worry that our selected definition of death will lead to treating persons who will not benefit. The case of retrieving organs presents a more interesting problem.

Prima facie, the higher brain definition of death would lead to the retrieval of more organs than say a whole brain or cardiopulmonary definition. The higher brain definition could justify taking organs from all those who can be justifiably used as donors under the whole brain definition plus all those who are in a persistent vegetative state. Those defending the cardiopulmonary definition risk losing transplantable organs, because the circulation of blood and oxygen preserves the organs. Once artificial respiration is withdrawn, physicians must move quickly to cool the organs to preserve them.

Whether different definitions of death will lead to significantly different numbers of retrieved organs is more complicated than first appears. A definition of death has consequences for retrieving organs, but the number of organs retrieved depends on other concepts, laws, policies, and technical strategies. We cannot expect or always desire that these strategies remain static so that definitions of death straightforwardly impact organ retrieval. The timing of declaring death will have an impact on organ retrieval, but only within a social context, one that functions within a conceptual and practical framework. Suggested and implemented adjustments with the cardiopulmonary definition of death illustrate the point.

6. The Cardiopulmonary Definition

In the light of problems with the whole brain and higher brain definitions, Truog advocates a return to the cardiopulmonary definition. Without making other adjustments, this move would lead to fewer organ transplants because waiting for the heart and lungs to stop functioning damages the deceased's organs. To compensate, Truog suggests that we abandon the Dead Donor Rule, a rule that prohibits retrieving organs from living persons whenever the procedure will kill the donor. Rejecting the Dead Donor Rule does not mean the transplant community would kill and retrieve organs from healthy living persons—they would only consider persons beyond the capacity for harm. Truog does not clarify his conception of harm the way Joel Feinberg does, but, presumably, he means that such donors would not be physically or psychologically hurt. He claims those we cannot possibly harm, "include those who are permanently and irreversibly unconscious such as patients in a persistent vegetative state or newborns with anencephaly and those who are imminently and irreversibly dying."[36]

Not shying away from controversy, Truog believes we ought to accept organ retrieval in the aforementioned cases as a form of justified killing. While this may send shock waves through many circles, he notes that many in medicine already implicitly accept this view. They do not believe that those who are brain dead are necessarily dead, and yet they feel justified in taking their organs. He adds that following principles of informed consent and nonmaleficence would guard against the slippery slope of creating an environment wherein transplant teams would prey upon vulnerable persons for their organs. He does believe that permitting the killing of seriously compromised persons for their organs may erode the value we place on life.[37]

Even if we reject Truog's suggestion, it shows that definitions of death only impact organ retrieval in concert with other practices. We can manipulate the number of organs retrieved in many ways.

Another way of demonstrating this point comes by way of retrieving organs from non-heart-beating cadavers. A famous instance, the Pittsburgh protocol approved in 1992, guides transplant teams in the retrieval of organs from patients who are not brain dead.[38] A committee at the University of Pittsburgh Medical Center designed the protocol to retrieve organs from patients on life support who want treatment withdrawn and who will die shortly thereafter.[39] When these patients declare that they want treatment withdrawn, physicians ask them whether they would like to donate their organs. If patients agree to donate, healthcare providers take them to the operating room where treatment is withdrawn. After withdrawing treatment from donors, clinicians wait for the absence of a pulse, apnea, unresponsiveness to verbal stimuli, and two minutes of ventricular fibrillation, asystole, or electromechanical dissociation.[40] When these conditions are satisfied, they retrieve the organs immediately. Since they are already in the operating room, they can cool the organs quickly for preservation.

The Pittsburgh protocol also shows the conceptual and technological adjustments people make to control the consequences of adopting a definition of death. Accepting the cardiopulmonary definition may not prevent the retrieval of as many organs as the whole brain definition, though it might not do as well as the higher brain definition in terms of organ retrieval. The Pittsburgh protocol also shows that healthcare providers do not actively care for patients while passively waiting for death—they determine the precise timing of death! For this reason, critics attack the Pittsburgh protocol on conceptual and moral grounds.

That physicians declare death two minutes after the patient's heart ceases, a time when physicians could resuscitate some of these patients, forms the core of conceptual criticism of the Pittsburgh protocol. It remains possible to reverse the deaths of these patients, but many persons believe that death is, by definition, irreversible.[41] David Cole claims that the Pittsburgh protocol interprets "irreversible cessation of cardiopulmonary function" as the low probability of auto-resuscitation. Cole does not find it odd to think we can bring a dead person back to life.[42]

In contrast, Tom Tomlinson interprets "irreversible" in a moral sense. In his view, "irreversible" means that the possibility of resuscitation is not morally significant. He reasons that with the Pittsburgh protocol the power to reverse death is not morally significant because patients agree to have treatment withdrawn and to donate.[43]

Regardless of our position on whether death is irreversible by definition, by fact, or neither, we still have room to argue over whether patients declared dead under the Pittsburgh protocol are, in fact, dead, and whether that is morally significant. Contrary to Cole and Tomlinson, Renee Fox says the Pittsburgh protocol is "the most elaborately macabre scheme" to retrieve organs. According to Fox, this practice subjects patients to an inhumane death because it takes them to the operating room to have treatment withdrawn.[44] This protocol means they die without the presence of their families. Fox thinks retrieving organs this way causes stress for the healthcare providers because patients die and have their organs removed on the same operating table—a powerful symbolic message that they are taking life to preserve a life.[44]

Bernat has also argued against the cardiopulmonary definition. He believes that irreversible loss of circulation is sufficient to define death, because irreversible loss of circulation leads to the death of all organs, including the brain.[45] He does not believe that the permanent loss of circulation is necessary for death. To demonstrate this point, he considers Alan Shewmon's gruesome but instructive thought experiment:

> Mr. A underwent surgical decapitation during which the major vessels of his head immediately were connected to a cardiopulmonary bypass machine permitting full and continuous preservation of brain functions. During the procedure, the body portion was attached to a mechanical ventilator permitting continuation of circulation to the neck, trunk, and limbs. Because the disconnected head portion contains a normally functioning brain, Mr. A retains the full capacity for awareness, thinking, experiencing, and communicating. In a second procedure, Mr. A's face and part of his skull, except his eyes, were grafted from the head portion onto the body portion. Mr. A's head portion continues to retain the full capacities of awareness, sentience, and communication.[46]

Bernat likes Shewmon's example because it shows that the head is alive, not the body, and he believes those who are declared brain dead according to whole brain standards are virtually identical to Mr. A.[47] The body is dead and circulation continues.

Bernat concludes that the loss of circulation is not necessary for death. He realizes that the example apparently fails to support his conclusion, because circulation continues within Mr. A's head. He counters that if an event destroyed the brain, and circulation continued, Mr. A would still be dead. In Bernat's words, "there seems no point in insisting that there is anything significant about the mere maintenance of circulation. All that is important is the continued functioning of the brain; when it is lost, the organism is dead."[48]

7. Conclusion

In summary, despite thirty years of debate, we still lack a compelling definition of death. We have seen that the higher brain, whole brain, and cardiopulmonary definitions all leave us with interesting and challenging questions. Small wonder, then, some persons have suggested that we decide among these definitions according to their moral consequences. I have emphasized that the moral consequences of each definition depend upon other practices that are subject to change. But which definition of death provides for the retrieval of the most organs all other things remaining equal? This question overlooks a central point of this book—many relevant practices, concepts, laws, and values are subject to change. The key question is what changes should be made?

We address this question by anticipating the moral features of adopting each definition only by considering a host of other possible adjustments. When we do so, we find that each definition will have both good and bad moral features and results; there will be losses and residue with each definition of death. The higher brain position contradicts many persons' intuitive understanding of death and may erode our respect for the lives of seriously compromised persons. Reverting to the cardiopulmonary position would seriously undermine the goals of transplantation, unless we also decide to abandon the Dead Donor Rule or find that we can retrieve many organs from those whose heart-lung function has ceased although their brains still function. But Bernat may be correct in thinking that rejecting the Dead Donor Rule would cause a backlash against organ retrieval and emphatically indicate a diminished respect for life.[49] The whole brain position appears to take a middle-of-the-road approach, even though many healthcare providers must believe the whole brain definition has led to the killing of severely compromised persons for their organs. Even if the whole brain definition is justifiable, I think it also undermines our respect for life and creates public distrust of the medical community.

Given the moral losses associated with each definition of death, we will need to examine ways to avoid or alleviate those losses. Can we find appropriate ways to retrieve more organs without relying upon dubious definitions of death and their undesirable moral consequences? Since the sources of organs here are the dead and the nearly dead, we cannot make amends to them for any moral losses resulting from adopting a definition of death. We can try to avoid conflicts, but it remains to be seen which conflicts we ought to avoid and how we should do so. In chapter ten, I address ethical issues related to avoiding conflicts. We must make choices, but the debate over the definition of death illustrates two significant problems when it comes to determining a single right answer to complex problems such as defining and declaring death.

The first problem is the incommensurability of values. No one has written a compelling account of how we should balance the conflicting values involved with the organ retrieval strategies discussed in this book. What we find in the literature are bold pronouncements by some scholars that other scholars find unconvincing. When moral issues are controversial, we need guidelines about comparing values or suggestions about what we should do in the light of imprecise or impossible value comparisons. The disagreements among scholars suggest that the incommensurability of values is part of the difficulty of developing a compelling case for a comprehensive organ retrieval strategy.

The second obstacle to determining a single right action is that we can manipulate the consequences of our choices in many ways. The definition of death illustrates the creative but sometimes disturbing efforts to yield more organs. At times, technological advances such as artificial respirators and conceptual changes in the meaning and criteria for death allow for the retrieval of more organs. Technological and conceptual changes require many of us to change psychologically as well. Can we convince ourselves that the higher brain or whole brain definitions adequately reflect our meaning of death? If not, can we convince ourselves that retrieving organs from severely compromised living persons is morally justifiable? Can we convince ourselves that the Pittsburg protocol is justified? And even if we make the needed psychological adjustments, are these conceptual and psychological adjustments morally justifiable?

The definition of death debate begins to show what I mean by constructive pluralism. First, we must recognize the plurality of values at stake in organ retrieval policies and practices, namely the respect for the sources of organs and the good of helping transplant candidates. Second, because we can manipulate the number of available transplantable organs in many ways, we must evaluate the adoption of a definition of death in the light of all other factors influencing the number of available organs. Third, due to conflicting values, adopting a definition will lead to good and bad moral results and controversies will continue. All the same, even those who advocate disturbing policies recognize the need to account for residue. This crucial commonality unites many who disagree over policies and practices. That is why Truog in advocating the retrieval of organs from persons barely alive also worries about eroding our respect for life. This explains why those who accept the Dead Donor Rule also believe we must find alternative retrieval practices and policies. The key, then, is to narrow the field of morally permissible options. In the next chapter, I discuss another alternative, the selling of organs.

Seven

THE SELLING OF ORGANS

The United States National Organ Transplant Act of 1984 (NOTA) prohibits "any person to knowingly acquire, receive, or otherwise transfer any human organ for valuable consideration for use in human transplantation, if the transfer affects interstate commerce."[1] NOTA precludes the direct sale of organs but permits fees paid to medical personnel, hospitals or other clinical services and reimbursements to donors for travel and housing expenses and for lost wages, and to donor recipients for legal or medical expenses.[2]

Regardless of NOTA's prohibition on sales, organ donors in Pennsylvania will have $300 paid toward their funeral expenses. Howard Nathan, president of the Gift of Life Donor Program, one of two centers that distribute organs in Pennsylvania, claims the initiative does not constitute the buying and selling of organs.[3] Instead, he says, "this is about having a voluntary death benefit for a family who gave a gift."[4] Not surprisingly, Jon Nelson of the Federal Health Resources and Services Administration believes federal law forbids the exchange of organs for any payment thereby implying the illegality of the Pennsylvania practice.[5] Whether the Pennsylvania initiative passes legal muster or leads to the retrieval of more organs will prove interesting. In this chapter, I explore the moral dimensions of selling organs.

The selling of organs conjures images of India's downtrodden selling a kidney for $1,000 to $1,500. Many Indians who sell a kidney feel degraded, but they are desperate. To make matters worse, the Indians who sell their organs remain poverty stricken.[6]

Purchasing organs need not be so obviously exploitive. As the Pennsylvania initiative indicates, we can restrict the retrieval of organs from living sellers (live-organ sales) while allowing financial benefits to sellers' families after sellers die (cadaveric organ sales). Even so, selling organs generates many practical and ethical questions. Is it likely that the sale of organs would significantly increase the organ supply? Would selling organs undercut respect for persons' bodies? Supposing that financial incentives would result in the retrieval of more organs, and that payments would undermine respect for persons, how should we respond to the conflict?

1. Financial Incentives and the Supply of Organs

Most of us probably assume that selling organs would increase the organ supply. One person who doubts this is John Walter Edinger.[7] As far as I know, Edinger's views have not been influential, but we should establish instead of assume that selling organs will increase the organ supply. I will critique three arguments that Edinger advances in his attempt to show that financial incentives are unlikely to increase the supply of transplantable organs.

One of Edinger's arguments stems from surveys that showed most people are willing to donate their organs but that United States healthcare providers are not asking families to consent to organ retrieval. From that, Edinger drew a plausible conclusion for the late 1980s; more awareness might obviate the need for financial incentives.[8] On the other hand, a study shows that United States healthcare providers frequently ask families to donate, but families often say no.[9] For this reason, Edinger's argument fails to show that financial incentives are not necessary.

In the second argument, Edinger claims that some donors under a voluntary system would decide not to donate under a combined voluntary-paid system.[10] He believes that persons could come to believe that a paid system obviates the need for voluntary donation. I doubt this would become an issue, though, since people motivated to donate their organs would still benefit themselves or their families by selling their organs. Edinger's worry pertains to those who would be primarily motivated for altruistic reasons who would also happen to believe the transplant community has obtained a sufficient number of organs. This possibility does not pose any problem that public announcements could not resolve.

In the third argument, Edinger addresses payments for organs made to a seller's family upon the seller's death. Edinger says that financial incentives would help relatives, but not the donors. His suppressed conclusion appears to be that if self-interest motivates people and if payments would go to the seller's family, then self-interested persons would not likely sell their organs since they would never reap any benefits. He reasons that sellers who would be motivated to help their families must have altruistic motives. If people are benevolent enough to sell their organs for the sake of their families, then they are probably sufficiently altruistic to donate their organs.[11] He presumes that many people who are willing to help their families would also help strangers.

Edinger's argument is not compelling. We often act benevolently toward family members where we would not for strangers. Self-interest dictates that selling our organs for the sake of our family may elicit rewards that donating our organs would not bring. Those willing to sell their organs may believe that family members will treat them with more respect and sensitivity, for instance. Maybe they will. If we take Pennsylvania's plan as a model, though, many family members would probably not treat organ sellers better for a mere $300. We cannot assume or infer from any of Edinger's considerations that financial incentives would fail to increase the organ supply.

Contra Edinger, financial incentives would probably increase the supply of organs. For one, among those who do not like the idea of donation, some will decide to sell their organs for the sake of financial benefit. Most of those who would altruistically donate their organs under our current system would still donate or sell their organs if we permitted organ sales. I do not see why permitting sales would discourage them from doing so. After all, would not many people consider it better to help others and receive pay for it? There would probably be fewer voluntary donors, but that is only because some former volunteers would decide to sell their organs. Some individuals might find financial benefits degrading, but I do not know how widespread this problem would be. Besides, they could refuse payment if they so desire. The Pennsylvania initiative will give us some indication as to whether small monetary incentives will help. We can assume that the greater the payment, the greater the increase in transplantable organs. Increasing the organ supply counts as a moral reason for permitting organ sales, but we must consider other issues before establishing the moral permissibility of organ sales.

2. Radin on Commodification

The apparent moral problem with organ sales is that something is wrong with selling one's body, that it morally diminishes everyone involved. Prostitution provides an obvious analogue, but so does the Marxist idea of selling one's labor for wages, especially meager wages. To decide the morality of organ sales, we must consider the extent to which persons should be free or autonomous to utilize their body. The issue over the moral permissibility of organ sales goes to the heart of what it means to be autonomous.

Classic liberals conceive of autonomy in terms of the absence of interference. Communitarians conceive of autonomy as having choices consistent with our highest aspirations of self-development in the context of a thriving, supportive community.[12] Regarding organ sales, we find this communitarian spirit manifested in three beliefs. We should seek to change our society if people feel the need to sell their organs; organ sales treat persons and their parts as mere commodities; and organ sales replace the deeply personal and altruistic value of giving another human being a part of oneself. We face the challenge, then, of reconciling organ sales with the views that people ought to control their bodies, that we should not allow the exploitation of poor persons, that people and their parts are not mere commodities, and that donating organs confers an altruistic value that organ sales cannot.

To explore these issues, I turn to Margaret Radin's exposition of commodification, the process and end of understanding something as a commodity.[13] I go on to discuss the ethics of retrieving a kidney, lung, or liver lobe from living sellers and then consider the ethics of selling cadaveric organs. I also examine the altruistic tradition of donating organs. Finally, I briefly discuss how we might establish payments for organ sellers.

For Radin, the central issue is whether allowing people to sell their organs enhances or compromises respect for them as persons deserving of dignified treatment. At one end of the spectrum, we have those who believe the marketplace allows persons to express their freedom and individuality.[14] On one radical view, liberals believe we can appropriately buy and sell all things, including organs.[15] On the other hand, we have Marxists who think all forms of commodification undermine respect for individuals.[16] In between, we have what Radin calls liberal compartmentalizers who seek to determine the proper scope of markets.[17]

Radin believes radical liberals, Marxists, and liberal compartmentalizers have all missed the mark. She rejects radical liberalism, because it conceives of people as mere commodity traders attempting to best satisfy their preferences in all circumstances. To her mind, we cannot exchange all values with money without some loss. A thing's market value does not constitute its total value. Nor does she think the radical liberal model fully captures what it means to be a person.[18] That is, we are not merely commodity traders. The Marxist position misses because markets have obviously been liberating to some extent.[19] Presumably, she means that free markets encourage persons to embark on projects, and people can freely exchange goods. She also rejects liberal compartmentalization, because restricting persons' freedom usually fails to respect them as persons as well.

As an alternative to the three aforementioned positions on markets, Radin defends what she calls incomplete commodification. She presumes that human interactions have overlapping meanings. In the context of discussing markets, she believes that an item can have a market value and an intrinsic value. For example, a painting can have a market value while its owner considers it priceless. Also, persons can work for money and find it meaningful.[20] The issue, then, is whether we can pay for people's organs, and still respect them.

Radin believes persons' willingness to sell their organs signals economic injustice, but says that even assuming that selling one's organs diminishes respect for persons, we do not cure the problem by prohibiting organ sales.[21] Instead, we should focus on the problems that give rise to such desperation. This does not mean she underestimates the problem of eroding respect for persons by permitting organ sales. In her words, "sale of one's body parts presents a dilemma because it seems we cannot honor our intuitions of what is required for society to respect personhood, either by permitting sales or by banning them."[22]

Although Radin makes no mention of the dilemmas debate previously discussed, her conception of a dilemma implicitly refers to the problem of inevitable moral loss and to the intuitive appeal of the regulative principle. Recall Ruth Charlotte Barcan Marcus's principle that we ought to restructure our lives with an eye toward avoiding conflicts. In Radin's words:

If neither commodification nor noncommodification can put to rest our disquiet about harm to personhood in conjunction with certain kinds of transactions, if neither commodification nor noncommodification can satisfy our aspirations for a society exhibiting equal respect for persons, then we must rethink the larger social context in which this dilemma is embedded.[23]

In an implicit appeal to the regulative principle she says, "if we agree that this dilemma means we ought to change the surrounding circumstances, we are still faced with the question of whether we should permit commodification while we try to do that."[24] In the final analysis, she believes we ought to permit the sale of organs, although she admits there is no algorithm for deciding the issue.[25] Unfortunately, Radin omits to clarify whether her arguments pertain to the sale of organs retrieved after a seller's death, or the retrieval of a kidney, lung, or liver lobe while the seller lives, or both. I will show that the ethics of live-organ sales differ from the ethics of cadaveric organ sales.

3. Live-Organ Sales and Respect for Persons

That live-organ sales leave sellers feeling diminished is not idle speculation. We should pay heed to the experiences of poor persons in India. In these cases, live-organ sales exploit persons' inability to earn money in ways that are more dignified. The feeling of diminution is not the only moral problem. Live-organ sales provide reflective persons with reasons for feeling devalued, because it inescapably treats them as a commodity, and it undermines the sanctity that we ought to have for persons' bodies. Live-organ sales disrespect the seller, and risk undermining the respect that we ought to have for all persons. We would know that in a community that permits live-organ sales, all persons' bodies are up for sale. Live-organ sales will also entice poor persons to do something that they would probably feel ambivalent about at best.

These considerations provide *prima facie* moral reason not to implement a system of live-organ sales. Recall that before concluding that live-organ sales is morally impermissible all things considered, we must evaluate the seller's autonomy, whether we prefer the liberal or communitarian conception of autonomy, and the impact of live-organ sales on organ retrieval. Whether the value of treating persons with respect overrides the value of honoring persons' right to make choices independently and the value of increasing the organ supply requires more thought.

Even when we acknowledge that live-organ sales disrespect persons, we should consider the autonomy of potential sellers. We must respect persons' right to make personal choices, especially when those choices involve the handling of their bodies. Putting everything up for sale is not morally permissible. Elizabeth Anderson points out, for instance, that we should not allow persons to sell their votes or to sell themselves into slavery. Doubtless, she could support her point on political and moral grounds. Similarly, although permitting live-organ sales shows respect for persons' right to choose, it fails to respect the sanctity of sellers' bodies. These points leave the issue indeterminate, so we must also consider the broader social impact of live-organ sales on retrieving more organs.

Whether live-organ sales are immoral, all-things-considered, depends to some extent upon the success of other retrieval strategies. Keep in mind that live-organ transplants are more successful than cadaveric transplants. If retrieving organs from living sellers is needed to extend the lives of many persons as part of a comprehensive approach to organ retrieval, we would have more reason to believe that live-organ sales is morally permissible. If selling cadaveric organs in conjunction with other organ retrieval strategies substantially increased the number of transplantable organs, live-organ sales would be more difficult to justify.

Although extending persons' lives is morally significant, we should create societies where we respect people and provide them with legitimate means to secure a comfortable standard of living. Since live-organ sales diminishes respect for persons, and we have other means to help those with failing organs, we have strong reasons to think live-organ sales are immoral all-things-considered as well. Many thoughtful readers may have contrary intuitions and views, especially since we Americans may sell our semen, eggs, hair, and blood.[26] Are these sales immoral as well?

I see no reason for thinking the selling of human hair is immoral, but I am inclined to think that selling blood, eggs, and semen is immoral when retrieved from living persons. For the same reason, buying organs from living persons is immoral; it treats persons disrespectfully by regarding their body parts as commodities. This view is difficult to defend, because whether a part of us is internal or external is not morally relevant. Nor can we plausibly argue that retrieving organs from living sellers is too risky. Even though withdrawing a kidney is more risky than withdrawing blood, we may take many sorts of risks for financial gain. As David Rothman states, "risk-conscious insurance companies do not raise their rates for kidney donors."[27]

Even though I cannot completely explain why I believe selling hair is morally permissible while selling blood, semen, and organs to be retrieved while the seller lives is immoral, I have given good reasons for thinking live-organ sales are immoral. My problem is that my account is incomplete in the sense that I do not have good reasons for all of my moral intuitions. Even if we can fortify the argument that live-organ sales are immoral all things considered, justifying the legal prohibition of live-organ sales requires additional evidence and considerations.

Many countries permit a variety of bodily insults, including actions that harm and disrespect participants and third parties. In the United States and other countries, we allow automobiles and petrochemical plants to spew toxins into our air. We allow corporations to feed us unhealthy food. Although we Americans prohibit prostitution, we allow peep shows and strip clubs. We pay lip service to opposing violence but we permit professional boxers, American football players, and hockey players to batter each other. We sound inconsistent at best and hypocritical at worst, if we say we want to prohibit live-organ sales on the basis that it undermines respect for persons.

Selling a kidney cannot be worse than allowing professional fighters to destroy each other's brains and kidneys, or allowing American football players to destroy each other's knees. I am not suggesting that we ban all activities that risk serious harm to participants or that treat persons disrespectfully, but the consistent application of values to ensure respect for persons without unduly intruding upon persons' autonomy is challenging.

I hope that all nations and the United States especially will not permit live-organ sales. We can approach organ retrieval in better ways without further diminishing respect for people's bodies. Understandably, though, some persons would advocate organ sales for the sake of extending persons' lives and of respecting persons' choices. If we did so, we would exploit the poor and disrespect persons in two senses. Live-organ sales disrespect the sellers and insidiously undermine respect for persons in general.

Some commentators have proposed ways to alleviate the losses from live-organ sales that reinforce justification of emphasizing adjustments made to create a justifiable balance of value. Even those who advocate retrieving kidneys from living sellers encourage the development of protective measures. Consider the following six proposals offered by Gloria J. Banks: (1) set a minimum sum for kidneys; (2) prohibit persons below a designated income from being sellers; (3) only allow federally licensed agencies to buy kidneys (4) impose a six-month waiting period between the signing of the contract and the retrieval of the kidney; permit sellers to rescind the agreement at any time; (5) require sellers to be at least twenty-five years of age; (6) require a physician and a social worker to examine candidate sellers, and a panel independent of the purchasing agency approves the sale.[28]

These six conditions set out to avoid exploiting the poor and other vulnerable persons. Even if we object to live-organ sales, these suggestions improve its moral position. Alleviating moral losses is part of a morally justifiable response. Although I will explore the issue further in chapter ten, all other things remaining equal, a response that alleviates or avoids moral losses is better than a response that fails to do so.

The one effect that these suggestions cannot alleviate is that such sales diminish respect for persons. We can also disrespect middle and upper class persons by permitting the purchase of their parts. Prohibiting the poor from being sellers might undermine the point of the policies—to retrieve many more organs. Why would many middle-class persons wish to sell a kidney?

This set of proposals raises two obvious objections—eliminating the poor from participating, and setting the age limit at twenty-five.

Ironically, the poor will never have the opportunity to make money by selling their organs, thereby avoiding exploitation. This proposal defies logic, for if we want to provide monetary rewards, we discriminate in the worst sense by excluding those who could most benefit. Would we also preclude the poor from donating their organs? Alternatively, would we allow the poor to donate but not sell their organs while wealthier persons may sell or donate their organs? In terms of treating the poor appropriately, an unblemished position is not possible. If we allow the poor to sell their organs, then we exploit them; if we allow everyone except the poor to sell their organs, we discriminate against them.

Addressing the age limit, only competent adults should decide to sell a kidney, lung, or liver lobe. The question is, when do individuals become competent adults? Any age set will be arbitrary, but setting the age at twenty-five sounds unjustified. Many teenage boys and girls have sacrificed their lives in wars, and the legal drinking age is twenty-one in the United States. Are we supposed to allow individuals between the ages of twenty-one and twenty-four to pickle their livers but not to sell them?

Unless someone offers justifiable reasons for having adulthood defined to begin at different ages, we should seek a consistent definition across policies. By setting legal or institutional age limits at eighteen, we could retrieve more organs. If allowing persons to sell their organs is not exploitive or disrespectful, why would we deprive mature individuals under twenty-five years of age of financial gain and the opportunity to save another person from premature death? On the other hand, if selling organs is exploitive or discriminatory, why should we encourage individuals of any age to sell their organs?

Just as developing a sense of community involves many variables, so does cultivating a society where we learn to treat persons and their bodies with respect. We should continue encouraging people to eat well, exercise, drink only in moderation, engage in respectful and fulfilling friendships and sexual relations, and avoid smoking and drug abuse. Refusing to allow live-organ sales should be a part of developing a society that respects persons beyond merely honoring their choices.

We Americans send many mixed messages about health, so it should not surprise us that many Americans indulge in unhealthy habits and have conflicting desires.

4. Cadaveric Organ Sales and the Altruistic Tradition

Radin correctly draws attention to social injustice that motivates people to sell their organs. We do not want people selling their kidneys to buy food and electricity for a few months, or for alcohol or drugs. This sort of exploitation would only be a problem for living persons who intend on selling a kidney or lobe from their liver or lung.

Thinking that we might financially exploit dead organ sellers who were poor if they gave prior consent is more controversial. Such thinking is not totally out of the question, though, since poor persons who have a strong aversion to donation could agree to sell their organs to pay off debts or to assist their poor relatives depending on the financial details. Such a decision could cause a person considerable anxiety about dying. There also remains a moral obstacle to paying for people's cadaveric organs: it transgresses the altruistic tradition of organ donation.

The altruistic tradition of organ donation means that people donate for the sake of helping those in need. Having an organ retrieval system based on altruism provides special meaning and value for donors and their families and for organ recipients. Since many donors are the victims of accidents, families feel that they can make something good of the tragedy by prolonging someone else's life. Recipients of organs feel a level of gratitude that will not occur if we allow the sale of organs. In a market for organs, transplant patients would still feel grateful for having their life extended, but their attitudes toward the donor must change. Do we not feel differently toward persons when they offer us gifts as opposed to when they sell us something? Organs are no different from other items in this respect. Gift giving warrants a respect and admiration that selling does not. Gift recipients participate in the benevolence of others and are touched and humbled in ways that cannot occur when selling organs. So, selling organs would result in diminishing the value achieved by donors and their families and the benevolence that benefits transplant patients under an altruistic system.

According to some scholars, though, not all is good with the gift relationship. Renee Fox and Judith Swazey have discussed the "tyranny of the gift."[29] To their minds, receipt of donated organs often burdens transplant recipients because they cannot possibly repay the donor. For this reason, an altruistic system has its negative aftermath as well. How then are we to balance the benefits and burdens of an altruistic system? Until someone provides us with detailed interviews with transplant recipients and their families regarding their feelings toward the donors, we will not be able to form accurate opinions. Whether the value of an altruistic system outweighs or takes priority over the aftermath from the "tyranny of the gift" appears to be one of those moral questions where our moral intuitions are inexact, thereby leaving us in need of broader theoretical concerns. But there may be other ways to justify cadaveric organ sales.

Supposedly, the value of an altruistic system consists in the strengthening of social bonds. Americans need a stronger sense of community, and an altruistic system helps the community in ways that retrieving organs after the seller's death does not. Yet, why should the burden of restoring communal bonds fall upon the organ retrieval and transplant industry? The organ re-trieval and transplantation industry is not the biggest factor in whether Ameri-cans live with a sense of community and common interests. All things consid-ered, permitting the sale of organs retrieved upon the seller's death may not further erode our communal bonds even though selling organs loses the aforementioned altruistic value between donors and recipients. This is so be-cause communal bonds strengthen through charitable involvement, commu-nity events, more direct political participation, and so forth. If we strength-ened communal bonds, there would probably be less need for any organ sales.

Until countries like the United States develop better approaches to pre-mature or congenital organ failure, the sale of cadaveric organs is justifiable. So long as sellers make an informed choice, the risk of wronging or harming the dead is negligible. In addition to contributing to the goals of transplanta-tion, we could also allow sellers to select a favorite charity as the beneficiary of the sale. While the sale of cadaveric organs partially undermines the altru-istic value of donation, the practice is justified for the sake of saving lives. But how would we implement an organ sales system?

5. Approaches to Selling Organs

Gloria Banks has succinctly summarized different approaches to establishing a commercial market in transplantable organs: a posthumous organ market, a living provider market, and a combined altruistic-commercial system.[30]

A posthumous organ market would allow payment to the donor, the de-ceased's estate, designee, or beneficiary upon death and the verification of transplantable organs.[31] This could work by either paying the seller upon fi-nalizing the contract or by paying the seller's family after the donor dies. Both approaches raise serious concerns. Paying the donor while alive would jeop-ardize the buyer's interest because the seller could damage his or her organs by smoking or drinking alcohol. The contract could include a provision for the seller to refrain from activities that would place the organs at risk, but en-forcement would be intrusive and impractical.[32] We can avoid these problems, if we make the payment after the seller's death.

Another option in the posthumous organ market would be to allow rela-tives of the decedent to sell the organs. In this case, organ retrieval organi-zations would solicit the decedent's family. We could provide families with the choice to donate or sell the organs, with any proceeds donated to their fa-vorite charity. Commentators have rightly pointed out that arranging such transactions would be awkward, potentially disturbing for the family, and im-practical due to time constraints.[33]

The best option would be to have payments for organs go to decedents' estates. Edmund Pellegrino fears that family members would precipitously re-quest the termination of treatment for organ sellers whose lives are in limbo.[37]

But this problem would be negligible. Physicians treating those at the end of life do not have to follow the wishes of the family if they believe withdrawing treatment violates the patient's best interest. We do not live in a perfect world, so there will be cases where organ sellers have their treatment ended prematurely, but we have no reason to think this would become a widespread problem. For this reason, the sale of organs when retrieved after the seller's death will not lead to the exploitation of many sellers.

6. Conclusion

In conclusion, I have argued for four main points. First, selling organs will probably increase the number of transplantable organs. Second, retrieving organs from living sellers violates respect for persons by treating them as a commodity and creates practical problems as well. Live-organ sales would insidiously diminish respect for people in general, if the practice became widespread. Third, retrieving organs from dead sellers is morally permissible, if sellers gave prior consent under reasonably fair conditions. Fourth, the best way to implement a system of cadaveric sales is to pay toward the decedent's funeral expenses or a charity. These arguments need strengthening, but this concession is consistent with what I say about how we ought to approach an overall strategy for helping those with failing organs.

At this point, I have discussed the ethics of routine retrieval, presumed consent, familial consent, defining death, and selling organs. In addition to the aforementioned problems of conflicting values, responding to residue, uncertainties regarding outcomes and the potential for scientific advancements, intuitions about the ethics of strategies vary among learned individuals. I am not the only person to admit to having weak intuitions about a policy—weak in the sense of not being confident in the correctness of the intuitions. Given the complexity of the issues and the lack of precise ethical tools when it comes to adjudicating conflicts, we should expect nothing less. The next two chapters address the most significant organ retrieval strategies: xenotransplantation, and stem cell research. Only these two strategies and routine retrieval raise the possibility of providing an inexhaustible supply of organs.

Eight

XENOGRAFTS

Xenografts or xenotransplants involve the transplantation of cells, tissues, or organs from a member of one species into an individual of another species. Transplants between closely related species are concordant; grafts between distantly related species, discordant. The transplantation of cells and tissues creates fewer medical problems than with whole organs. Immediate rejection of whole organs is more likely to occur with discordant grafts than with concordant transplants.[1]

Cross-species transplantation has been done for centuries. Only in recent decades have scientists provided good reasons for considering cross-species transplantation as a viable option for transplant candidates. Several developments have fostered hope: success with the xenotransplantation of cells and tissues such as porcine heart valves, improved immunosuppressants, the development of transgenic swine, and the more limited goal of using animal organs as bridges until we can find suitable human organs. In what follows, I summarize the history of xenotransplants, describe current developments, and explore two ethical issues—the ethical treatment of non-human animals and the risk of transmitting diseases to third parties. I support the transplantation of animal cells and tissues into human beings, but I do not argue for the point. I do support a moratorium on the xenotransplantation of whole organs. Hereafter, when I speak of xenotransplants I am referring to whole organ transplants unless otherwise specified.

1. Historical Background

Xenotransplants began in the seventeenth century. After William Harvey's demonstration of heart function and blood circulation, Richard Lower transfused the blood of a lamb into a man in 1667. He chose a lamb for its symbolic affiliation with Jesus of Nazareth.[2] In England, in the nineteenth century, physicians transferred sheep's blood into wayward husbands, those inclined toward violence, and general troublemakers.[3] Fortunately, the obstetrician James Blundell discovered the incompatibility of heterologous blood after conducting experiments with transfusing sheep blood into dogs, and the further development of xenografts was discouraged after Henry Gradle's failed transfusion of lamb's blood into a tubercular patient.[4] Still, medics transferred sheep blood into wounded soldiers during World War I.[5]

In the 1920s the Russian surgeon Serge Voronoff performed over fifty testicular transplants from apes and monkeys into men. Voronoff claimed that his patients were rejuvenated, but since no form of immunosuppressive drugs were available, the transplanted tissue did not probably survive for more than a few days. Vornoff was so convinced that monkeys would provide a surplus of parts for human beings that he established a farm to breed monkeys.[6]

In the early twentieth century, several breakthroughs such as Joseph Lister's production of antisepsis and Karl Landsteiner's discovery of chemical reactions with blood incompatibility stimulated transplantation advances.[7] In 1912, the French physician Alexis Carrel won the Nobel Prize in Physiology and Medicine for developing surgical techniques for joining blood vessels with organ transplantation in mind. Carrel also suggested that pigs might provide us with needed organs in the future.[8] In 1923, Carlos Williamson arrived at a basic understanding of organ rejection in which the immune system differentiates one's self from foreign tissue; in the 1950s Emile Holman learned about the role of antibodies in rejection; and in 1960 MacFarlane Burnet and Peter Medawar received the Nobel Prize for studies on animals' ability to tolerate foreign bodies.[9] Predictably, surgeons pursued xenotransplantation more enthusiastically in the 1960s.

In 1963, Claude Hitchcock transplanted into a sixty-five-year old woman a baboon kidney that functioned for four days. Shortly thereafter Keith Reemtsma and Thomas Starzl performed several transplants from chimpanzees and baboons. They chose primates because of their genetic similarity to human beings. Starzl's patients functioned without dialysis for ten to sixty days, and one of Reemtsma's transplants worked for nine months. In 1964, James D. Hardy transplanted a chimpanzee heart into a sixty-eight-year old man, the first heart xenograft. The heart functioned for only two hours. In the late 1960s, Starzl performed several transplants involving chimpanzee livers. The most successful patient survived nine days. Despite the poor results, Medawar claimed, "we are achieving greater success with grafts between species today than we achieved with grafts within species fifteen years ago. We will solve the problem of using heterografts one day if we try hard enough, and maybe in less than fifteen years."[10]

Rebecca Malouin points out the irony of Medawar's claim, since nearly fifteen years later, in 1984, the case of "Baby Fae" cast a dark cloud over the world of xenotransplantation.[11] Dr. Leonard Bailey of Loma Linda University transplanted a baboon's heart into "Baby Fae," who had a lethal heart problem. "Baby Fae" died three weeks after the surgery.[12] "Baby Fae" was doomed because of the lack of effective immunosuppressive drugs. Making matters worse, "Baby Fae's" blood type was O and baboons only have A, B, and AB blood types.[13]

The public, news commentators, and bioethicists condemned the transplant, because the child had little opportunity to benefit from the surgery. They accused Dr. Bailey of experimenting on a baby and of going to egregious lengths to promote himself as a leading surgeon. Despite the case's notoriety, Peter Singer points out that in 1987 the American National Institutes of Health agreed to contribute $3.36 million to the Columbia Presbyterian Medical Center in New York for research on transplanting chimpanzee hearts into human beings.[14]

In the 1990s, several developments increased enthusiasm for xenotransplants. Xenografts of tissues and cells can help patients with Parkinson's disease, muscular dystrophy, and diabetes by stabilizing insulin levels. The transplantation of tissues and cells from other animals to humans is not as prone to rejection as is the transplantation of whole organs. Ingenious methods for preventing rejection have proven successful. One technique involves enclosing animal cells and tissues within porous tubes or spheres that permit substances such as insulin to pass through but prevent the passage of immune system cells or antibodies that would cause rejection.[15] Harold Vanderpool reports that one company has transplanted transgenic pig organs into non-human primates with a less than 2 percent hyperacute rejection rate. Researchers predict that pig hearts, kidneys, and lungs will be able to function in human beings.[16]

Transplant surgeons considered baboons as a potential source of organs, but the use of baboons runs into practical and moral problems. Baboons take five to seven years to reach sexual maturity and are costly in terms of time and the money needed to take care of them. Estimates indicate that it would take seven to ten years and eight to ten million dollars to create 100 baboons free of identified pathogens.[17] Primate intelligence also makes using them for the benefit of human beings difficult to justify.

The Committee on Xenograft Transplantation believes pigs would provide a more feasible and morally defensible option. Pigs reach sexual maturity in six months and have only a four-month gestation period. Pigs can also produce two litters a year that yield from three to thirteen piglets, and they grow quickly; within three to six months their organs are large enough to transplant into adult human beings.[18]

Scientists also have information regarding pigs' tissue types and they have bred pigs to have type O blood that is compatible with all types of human blood. Scientists have identified the exact target of antibodies that attack the transplanted pig organ, a sugar molecule abbreviated as Gal, which is a form of galactose. Currently, scientists are developing methods to remove anti-Gal antibodies from the transplant candidate and to engineer pigs that no longer express Gal.[19]

The Committee claims pigs provide a better moral choice than primates do because many human beings eat pork.[20] The Committee must mean that using pigs is less likely to trouble individuals. True, but that does not give us insight as to whether we ought to use pigs for transplantation. Even if it would be morally better to use pigs instead of baboons, we still must decide whether we ought to use pigs. Most people believe that we ought to utilize many animals for human purposes, but we need a moral justification.

2. Qualitative Distinctions and Human Privilege

Ray G. Frey has set out a philosophical defense of the use of animals in medical experimentation and treatment for the sake of human beings.[21] Although Frey does not tailor his argument for application to xenotransplants, he explicitly includes xenotransplants as a technology that his argument seeks to justify. While Frey believes the lives and experiences of all sentient creatures have value, he thinks we have good grounds for valuing humans over other animals. Frey's crucial premise is that humans' quality of life is vastly richer than that of other animals, including primates. In Frey's words:

> While we share many activities with animals, such as eating, sleeping, and reproducing, no combination of such activities comes anywhere near exhausting the richness of normal adult human life, where love, family, friends, art, music, literature, science, and the further products of reason and reflection add immeasurably to our lives. Moreover, and this is the point, we can mold and shape our lives in ways that are themselves additional sources of value; we can live out the lives of academic, artist, or ballplayer . . . we are creatures that can fashion our lives in order best to suit how we want to live.[22]

He concludes that a conflict between saving the lives of human beings and other animals should be resolved by saving human beings.

Animals such as pigs and baboons have valuable experiences, but I agree that experiencing complex emotions and thoughts is more valuable than physical pleasures and pains that we share with animals. In some circumstances we ought to save a human being over another sort of animal.

Frey recounts a case that appeared in a Florida newspaper in which the owners of a yacht had to choose between their dog and a crewmember when the yacht sank.[23] They chose the dog. The man died. I agree with Frey that the couple made the wrong choice. This intuition suggests that dogs are not as valuable as human beings are. If we substitute a pig for the dog—and I have heard that pigs are smarter than dogs and affectionate too—they should save the man without hesitation. Whether it would be immoral to choose Coco the gorilla over another human being, especially a despicable human being, say, a serial killer is murky. Still, I think most human beings should take priority over Coco, but the more we learn about animals, the more we realize that many species do have complex emotions and thoughts.

In what follows, I give reason to pause before accepting Frey's contention that if there are qualitative distinctions among animals' experiences, then we can justifiably sacrifice those animals lower on the scale for those that rank higher.

Attention to qualitative distinctions in experience inevitably leads us to question qualitative distinctions among human beings, even so-called normal human beings. If Frey is right that qualitative distinctions in our experiences determine our moral worth, and if qualitative distinctions exist among so-called normal human beings, it follows that some so-called normal human beings are more morally worthy than others unless reaching an identified threshold makes an individual inviolable. With this in mind, I focus on slippery-slope arguments that show Frey's argument can lead to absurd results.

Before adducing my slippery-slope argument, I will present two others. Jonathan Hughes has clarified the first one. Hughes's first premise is that different human beings have different intellectual and emotional capacities. To the extent that living a valuable life is a function of cognitive-emotional abilities, not all humans experience or create the same level of value. Examples abound—anencephalic infants, the severely retarded, many seriously ill patients, comatose persons, and those in a persistent vegetative state do not have lives as valuable as those of most normal human beings. Hughes believes that Frey's view entails that it would also be permissible to extract organs from the seriously mentally challenged for the sake of normal functioning humans. If we are uncomfortable with this conclusion, Hughes adds that consistency demands we should cease such experimentation on animals.[24]

Some species have more complex mental and emotional lives than those who are severely retarded. Although Hughes does not push the point, if he is right about Frey's account, then it would follow that severely debilitated humans could have their organs justifiably taken for the sake of primates and pigs, assuming that no normal functioning human being was in need of a transplant.

An obvious strategy that Frey might take to block Hughes's argument would be to rely on another slippery-slope argument. Frey could say that sacrificing severely debilitated persons would create social outrage and be impermissible on utilitarian grounds. Frey says that opposing the use of some human beings such as anencephalic infants for organ transplants because it would create social unrest is not convincing; people's attitudes can adjust to new practices. Frey might accept this strategy to undermine Hughes's criticism of his own argument, since the use of anencephalic infants is far less controversial than killing conscious but seriously limited human beings. At any rate, Frey does not introduce such arguments to support his cause, and doing so might not be consistent.

Frey believes we ought to use seriously impaired individuals for the benefit of human beings with normal mental capacities.[25] He recommends that we use anencephalic infants for organ transplants, an option that the American Medical Association supported in 1995 but later retracted. Although some reason exists for thinking we ought to use anencephalic infants and persons in a persistent vegetative state as organ donors, I have more difficulty thinking that we ought to use severely mentally handicapped individuals this way.

I do not know what Frey thinks about these options, but I believe he would want to avoid that consequence. Interestingly, though, after discussing the use of anencephalic infants as a source of organs, Frey uses the word "human" instead of "anencephalics" when arguing that human beings sometimes have less rich experiences than animals have, and that we should use human beings for scientific and medical purposes. Anencephalic infants are human beings, but either Frey sought to avoid repetitively using "anencephalics" or he means his argument to apply to several sorts of human beings who have a poor quality of life or no quality at all. Where would Frey want to draw the line related to the sacrifice of human beings for medical progress?

To better appreciate the problems with Frey's argument, I will consider one more slippery-slope argument. If Frey is right, it must also be true that even among human beings who have normal mental function those with richer emotions, thoughts, and projects are more valuable than persons whose sentiments, thoughts, and projects will always or usually be unrefined. This follows unless we identify a threshold of inviolability.

Some persons have richer friendships and amorous relationships, a deeper understanding of the value of art, philosophy, and the sciences, a better appreciation of music, food and beverages, nature, and their occupations and avocations. Some individuals have a greater ability to create valuable projects and enrich other people's lives than do others. Self-reflection shows that even an individual's moral, aesthetic, and rational sensibilities vary at times. Overall, among normally functioning humans, some people lead lives with more valuable experiences and projects than others do. On Frey's account, some normal individuals would be more valuable to save than other normal people, resulting in an absurdity. In principle, it would be justifiable to kill some normal individuals for the sake of others. For this reason, we must pause before accepting Frey's highly intuitive premise that quality of life is a factor in an individual's moral worth. Let us consider how someone might try to undermine my argument.

To avoid the slippery slope to which I believe Frey leads us, we could say that determining which persons have richer experiences, emotions, thoughts, and projects is impractical. We could never be justified in deciding that we should sacrifice one human being with normal mental abilities for another, even if we accept Frey's premise that moral worth varies with the quality of a life. We could say that we can never, or virtually never, justifiably kill any individual who reaches a designated cognitive-emotional threshold and ability for creating a valuable life for the sake of another individual. All human beings with normal mental functioning meet or surpass that threshold. Finally, we could say that such sacrifices would cause a social uproar.

Although all of these responses to my slippery-slope argument are plausible, none accomplishes what we need from moral arguments. Frey would want, I think, a way to justify utilizing animals scientifically and medically including for xenotransplants without leading to absurd results such as allowing and even encouraging sacrificing some normally functioning human beings for the sake of those who have richer and more valuable lives. The problem with the first argument is that the epistemological problem of determining which individuals live richer lives is not the only or primary reason why we ought to refrain from sacrificing normal persons. Otherwise, we would be committed to accept as true the following conditional statement: if it were possible to determine which individuals experience valuable lives, then we could justifiably sacrifice those individuals who lead inferior lives. The problem is not merely that we lack the knowledge of who to sacrifice; sacrificing normal persons for those with superior lives is immoral in principle.

Let us consider whether meeting a designated threshold makes an individual inviolable. Perhaps it does. The problem, though, is that the threshold argument invites disputation over the appropriate threshold. Animal rights activists can agree that such a threshold exists, but deny that it begins with human beings with normal mental capacities. Primates apparently experience love, sorrow, and jealousy.[26] Why not draw the line earlier with sentience or at a lower level of intelligence? Frey's argument cannot support xenografts without defending a threshold of inviolability that animals used for medical research fail to meet but normal functioning human beings meet or surpass.

The third argument is open to the same sort of objection as the first argument. We should not think that the best reason for not sacrificing one human being for the sake of another human is to prevent social chaos. I suspect that Frey would agree. I do not see how Frey can give us good reasons for refraining from sacrificing a normal human being for an aesthete who relishes life and who creates many valuable projects that benefit many others. Again, the problem is not merely that this would upset the social order; doing so is wrongheaded in principle.

With Frey, I believe that most human lives are more valuable than most animals' lives. I also agree with Frey that qualitative distinctions among candidates for, or bearers of, moral status are relevant for applied ethics. Unlike Frey, I am not convinced we have found good reason to believe that we may justifiably sacrifice the lives of all types of animals for human lives. Nor am I in a good position to develop an argument as to where we should draw a threshold line. Recall Tom Beauchamp and James Childress's admonition that our moral beliefs will likely contain some inconsistencies. Although inconsistency is not inevitable, many highly intuitive moral beliefs do lead to inconsistencies or counter-intuitive results. With that reminder, I turn to the second significant problem for defenders of xenotransplants—risks to third parties.

3. Risks to Third Parties

Xenografts present medical risks to third parties. Microorganisms that are benign in one species can be fatal to another. B virus usually does not cause disease in the macaque monkey but can cause serious neurological damage to human beings—enough to cause a 70 percent mortality rate. We know that pigs carry pseudorabies virus and baboons carry foamy virus, but do not know whether these viruses will create diseases in humans. Examples abound where a virus transmitted to one person eventually infected many others. In 1967, in Germany, vervet monkeys transmitted the Marburg virus to thirty-one persons. In a more startling case, a single person admitted into a hospital in Zaire in 1976 with Ebola hemorrhagic fever (EHF), caused by the Ebola virus, infected over two hundred persons and eighty-eight percent of them died.[27]

Retroviruses such as HIV generate more serious worries about public health because they have a long latency period.[28] This means that a retrovirus transmitted from an animal to the transplant patient could then infect several other persons before symptoms appeared, and before anyone could identify the problem. Only recently have scientists learned that porcine endogenous retroviruses can infect human cells.[29] Consequently, Jonathon Allan organized a letter signed by forty-four scientists declaring that supporters of xenotransplants have not adequately addressed infectious disease concerns.[30]

Does the potential good of xenotransplantation outweigh the possible harm? According to Harold Vanderpool, researchers are finding that infection from porcine endogenous retrovirus may have been overestimated.[31] Unfortunately, we cannot perform a precise cost-benefit analysis. As the Committee on Xenograft Transplantation recognized, we cannot identify all of the hazards, because animals will probably possess unidentified viruses that might be harmful to humans.[32] Even when scientists identify viruses, we do not always know whether they will prove harmful to human beings. The Committee concluded, "risk management depends on professional judgment, and the public should be informed that the management plan represents a best guess for minimizing risks."[33] In their judgment, not proceeding with xenotransplant research would diminish our humanity.[34]

4. The Prospects of Xenografts

Despite the harm to animals and the potential problems with transmitting diseases to patients and third parties, the push to develop xenografts will likely increase. Powerful forces have an intellectual and financial interest in their development. Abdallah Salim Daar has pointed out that several companies have collaborated with academic institutions to perform research. Biotransplants and Cell Genesys are working with Harvard, and Imutran is working with Cambridge University. As Daar notes, these companies will likely lobby to accelerate xenotransplants to recover their investment and establish their technology. Unfortunately, the companies will likely be reluctant to share their data and will probably insist that physicians under contract keep the information confidential.[35]

Although we should not take the development of xenotransplants to be inevitable, we ought to anticipate with as much detail as possible what life with widespread xenotransplants would be like. We do not know for sure what xenotransplants would bring, but Daar has identified some plausible consequences and likely required adjustments. He has spelled out residual reasons and requirements we would have if we pursued xenotransplantation.

According to Daar, we would have to strictly monitor and perhaps quarantine early recipients. Due to the risk to third parties, he believes we would need to secure community consent through public hearings, advisory boards, and legislation. Prolonged monitoring of the patient would transform informed consent into something more like a contract, a contract that could be intrusive to the point of requiring patients not to have sexual relations for up to a year. He also says that xenotransplantation would contribute to a shift from the altruistic donation of organs to a market in organs.[36]

Presumably, this shift would occur because biotechnology companies will have the legal right to many products of xenotransplant research. Genetically engineered pigs cannot donate their organs, and if these organs prove effective, then the need for human donation would vanish. Daar believes that if we permit xenografts, the practice will probably serve only as a bridge until we can find human organs. This fact would increase the pressure to employ other means of organ retrieval such as a presumed consent law and to permit the buying and selling of organs. Along with others, Daar believes that xenotransplantation will undermine human beings' willingness to donate their organs due to disgust, fear, and distrust of technology, and the perception that people no longer need to donate.[37]

We cannot be sure that all of Daar's predictions will materialize, but he offers us crucial issues to consider. Whatever we decide as individual nations and as a global community, there will be moral losses from our decisions and new conflicts will emerge. To develop xenografts means creating risks to third parties and the destruction of pigs. Refraining from performing xenotransplants of whole organs would not result in the loss of more human lives at the present; yet, a moratorium will truncate the growth of knowledge that could significantly prolong the lives of many persons in the future. Although I believe human beings are more valuable than pigs, I also believe we should place a moratorium on the xenotransplantation of whole organs for two principal reasons. First, the likelihood of transmitting diseases to the community is too great a risk. Second, we can pursue other options to benefit transplant candidates—a point that I will further discuss in chapter nine.

5. Conclusion

In conclusion, history reveals a dismal record of xenotransplantation. Transplant surgeons are notorious for their misleading optimism, but recent developments have renewed faith in the procedure. Although morality dictates that we do something to help those with failing organs, xenotransplants present too great a risk to the community. I have also argued that one enticing argument to justify the killing of animals for humans is problematic. Since I object to xenotransplants, I face the challenge of finding other ways to help those in need of a transplant.

We need better moral concepts. The plausible view that the level of moral concern depends upon a human being's ability to experience higher levels of value leads to troublesome results. It shows that we need a standard of moral inviolability if we are to accept the premise that the degree of moral concern hinges upon an individual's quality of experiences and projects. Whether we look for a moral discovery or encourage the construction of better moral concepts, the point is that we need better moral concepts. To help bring this about, we need better communication between ethical theorists and applied ethicists in medicine. In the next chapter, I will explore another strategy to help transplant candidates—stem cell research.

Nine

STEM CELL RESEARCH

Stem cells possess the ability to generate a line of identical cells for long periods of time and to differentiate into other types of cells.[1] These abilities support the long-term fantasy that the cells can develop into whole organs such as hearts, livers, and kidneys that surgeons can then transplant. More realistically, stem cells can restore health by regenerating damaged tissue when injected into failing organs.[2]

Most stem cell research is not controversial because scientists derive the cells from mice, placentas, fetal tissue obtained from miscarriages, human fat, and adult cells.[3] Controversy arises with embryonic stem cells that are isolated by separating a mass of cells that would have developed into the placenta and fetus. The outer layer of cells that would become the placenta—the blastocyst—is dissolved; the leftover mass that would become the fetus is used for research.[4] Scientists also derive embryonic stem cells from the gonadal tissue of aborted fetuses or the inner mass of blastocysts taken from embryos donated by parents who sought *in-vitro* fertilization treatment.[5] Until recently, people believed that adult stem cells were less capable than embryonic stem cells of developing into different cell types, thereby lending credence for the need for embryonic research. New studies indicate that adult stem cells are more flexible than previously thought, suggesting that embryonic research is unnecessary.[6] Such research is relatively new. Banning or severely limiting such research is difficult to justify.

1. United States Policy

In 1996, the United States Congress banned federal funding for any research that harms or destroys human embryos, but using federal funds to derive and use stem cells from donated fetal tissue is legal.[7] The fetuses are already dead, so the derivation of stem cells cannot cause the fetus's death. Presumably, stem cell research cannot cause harm to dead fetuses either. Otherwise, any federal funding for stem cell research would be illegal. While we continue to debate the moral status of living and dead embryos and fetuses, private firms like the Geron Corporation may produce stem cells for profit. Not surprisingly, discussion of the ethics of stem cell research has intensified.

In December of 1998 Harold Varmus, National Institutes of Health (NIH) director, requested an opinion on the legality of research funded by the NIH. In January of 1999 the general counsel of the Department of Health and Human Services (DHHS), Harriet S. Rabb, ruled that the NIH may legally fund uses of stem cell research but could not fund the derivation of stem cells from embryos. The reason is that the derivation process kills the embryo. Since stem cells are not embryos, the statute does not prevent NIH from funding stem cell research if scientists derived the stem cells from privately funded research. Rabb also interpreted federal law to permit the NIH to support the derivation and use of stem cells taken from fetal tissue.[8] Seventy-three eminent scientists, including sixty-seven Nobel Prize recipients, signed a letter supporting the NIH's consideration to finance research with stem cells originating from human embryos.[9]

On 9 August 2001, President George Walker Bush announced that federal funds may be utilized for stem cell research under the following conditions: research is performed on the sixty stem cell lines already developed; the embryo from which the stem cell line was derived cannot become a human being; the stem cells were derived from embryos created for reproductive purposes; the embryo is no longer needed for reproductive purposes; informed consent was obtained for the donated embryo; and no monies are provided for the donated embryos. Bush pledged that the government would spend $250 million on stem cell research for that year alone. This decision allowed Bush to permit crucial research without alienating pro-life supporters by sanctioning the destruction of embryonic human life. Our challenge is to determine the moral status of embryonic stem cell research, especially in light of new studies supporting the research potential of adult stem cells. This debate has benefited from a report from the Geron Corporation.

While Geron Corporation conducted stem cell research, they convened the Geron Ethics Advisory Board (EAB), an independent group of bioethics scholars assigned to evaluate and review the ethics of the company's stem cell program. The EAB unanimously agreed to six principles, the first of which is especially significant for our discussion of the quest for organs: embryonic tissue, including the blastocyst, deserves respect.[10] In what follows, I will explore the moral dimensions of this principle.

2. The Moral Status of Early Human Life Forms

When deliberating whether the blastocyst deserves moral consideration, the committee considered three schools of thought. The genetic school believes moral consideration begins at human conception. The social consequence school believes socially constructed norms, not biological facts, determine an entity's moral status. The EAB endorsed the developmental school: the view that human life begins at conception but moral status progressively grows with biological and cognitive development. The EAB accepted birth as the moment of full moral consideration—presumably that level of moral regard owed to human beings that does not increase with further cognitive and biological development.[11] Many find the developmental position appealing, but it does have its critics.

Glenn McGee and the prominent bioethicist Arthur Caplan do not believe appealing to biological development decides the moral status of embryonic cells. Instead, they adopt a version of the social consequence school. According to them, the meaning—read ascribed moral status—that we attach to cells depends upon the institutional context. They point out that the law treats frozen sperm as property in divorce settlements; agencies make frozen embryos available for adoption; and cloning enables skin cells to become embryos. Likewise, the moral status of fetuses depends on the technological ability to successfully deliver them at different stages of development.[12]

American social practices, including court rulings, the adoption of embryos, and our consideration of fetuses in early stages of development, indicate that embryos, fetuses, and even sperm possess considerable moral importance in some contexts. According to McGee and Caplan's understanding, if the developmental school is correct, embryos, sperm, early-stage fetuses, and skin cells either have no or little *intrinsic* moral status. McGee and Caplan presuppose that if the moral status of an entity changes with technological advancements or changing social contexts, then the moral status cannot be merely a matter of biological development.

We must wonder what McGee and Caplan think they have shown. Is it that biological and cognitive development is not sufficient to establish an entity's moral status, or that biological and cognitive development is not necessary? Alternatively, is such development one factor among many that determine an entity's moral status? All of the above? In light of McGee and Caplan's criticism, it may appear to us that biological development is merely one morally relevant factor among many; technological abilities and institutional contexts would be others. Although true, the point needs qualification.

If Sophie had to choose between one of her children and a blastocyst, embryo, or fetus, her choice ought to be much easier. The institutional context or level of available technology would count little, if at all. Even if such a decision would be psychologically difficult—no apparent dilemma exists between a blastocyst and a grade school child smart enough to play the violin, as is the case with Sophie's daughter.

Could there be a conflict between a child and a blastocyst? Yes, but one easily resolved. If we accept that blastocysts, embryos, and fetuses deserve moral consideration, the cognitive and emotional sophistication of a child means that children are more valuable than blastocysts, embryos, and fetuses. The best explanation for this revised Sophie's choice is that biological development counts a lot. There appears to be some truth to Frey's contention that the qualitative level of experience is relevant for our moral deliberations.

What we need, then, is a way to accommodate McGee and Caplan's insights with those of the developmental school. Fortunately, a straightforward answer exists. The reason the moral status of a given entity such as a blastocyst or an embryo changes according to context is that the moral factors change as well. A couple's infertility troubles provide moral reasons to care for their blastocysts. That is also true of any couple who wants children—caring for their sperm, eggs, zygotes, embryos, and fetuses has value in virtue of the value of having and caring for children. At the same time, biological and cognitive development sets limits as to what is morally permissible or required across contexts.

Abortion remains controversial, but parents do not have the right to kill toddlers. Advocates of the developmental position can say that couples benefiting from in vitro fertilization do not have a requirement to decide that each of their embryos develops into a well-functioning human being. The selection of an embryo to become the couple's child requires everyone involved to meet minimal professional and parental standards to protect the developing embryo. The context of IVF that incorporates the prospective parents' goals changes the value of embryos, but we have reason to think the level of biological and cognitive development of embryos makes them expendable whereas children are not. We can reject the developmental position based on the inviolability of all human life (genetic school), but the developmental school is not incoherent or fundamentally mistaken as McGee and Caplan suggest.

I agree with the EAB that blastocysts and embryos do not deserve the moral protections accorded to most human beings. Still, the EAB believes the blastocyst has some moral status.[13] To what extent do blastocysts deserve moral respect? Since the blastocyst does not have sensation, requirements to minimize pain or maximize pleasure do not apply. The EAB's answer is, "early embryonic tissue is respected by ensuring that it is used with care only in research that incorporates substantive values such as reduction of human suffering."[14] I take it that they mean researchers must aim to minimize suffering for sentient and rational beings, presumably human beings but perhaps other animals as well. As Lori P. Knowles notes, what they mean by "incorporates substantive values" is vague.[15] She fears that such weak language will permit The Geron Corporation to justify any research.

The EAB helps specify its meaning by claiming that researchers must treat utilized tissues with respect by taking into account families' needs for closure, grief, rituals, and respectful handling. Research requires informed consent.[16] I think the EAB gets the main issues right. That is, in virtue of being a living thing and, perhaps, having symbolic value, embryos and fetuses have some moral status, but the importance of biomedical research, including the desire to renew organs, justifies stem cell research.

3. Property Rights

Knowles and Gladys White rightly state that the most significant moral problems with stem cell research involve the rights of private corporations to own the stem cells and their potential to monopolize scientific knowledge. Knowles asks whether the corporation conducting the research or the parents possess legal rights to the stem cells. Answering this question will have moral import. Knowles says that allowing companies to patent a cell line gives them authority to restrict licensing of those cells according to their standards. Allowing patents also allows the companies to control access to their information and use of the cells in a way that can restrict the dissemination of scientific knowledge. Private ownership has the potential to curtail the alleviation of human suffering. Knowles understands the conflict: private funding for medical research could dry up without the ability to develop profitable patents. Like Margaret Radin, Knowles believes we can promote profits and altruism: we can praise couples who donate, allow companies to profit, and make medical benefits of the research available to all those in need. In her words:

> this means regulating the patent process so that others have access to the cells for further research and so that the pricing of products does not necessarily exclude those within or beyond our national borders who cannot afford expensive treatments.[17]

To accommodate these values, Knowles believes we must acknowledge that the American legal system needs changing. Knowles does not give us details regarding the needed changes, but she does say that we need to create special rules to include atypical sorts of property such as frozen embryos and stem cells.[18] We can and should make these changes, but we will need guidelines until those changes come to fruition.

White believes that for the immediate future we should plan to derive stem cells from fetal tissue instead of embryos. Her reasons are practical. The use of fetal tissue is far less contentious than utilizing embryos.[19] The reason is that deriving stem cells from embryos requires killing them.

As John Fletcher notes, unless we think embryos have no moral status, research on embryos will be more controversial than research with fetuses. If killing embryos is immoral, even for research purposes, then the issue arises whether we may use stem cells derived from immoral means.[20] In addition, there remain unanswered questions as to how we are to acquire spare embryos. Will women or couples donate spare embryos from *in-vitro* fertilization (IVF) clinics? Or will scientists develop stem cells from donated egg and sperm cells?[21] We can avoid many of these moral issues if adult stem cells prove as efficacious as embryonic stem cells.

4. Adult Stem Cells

Recent research shows that adult stem cells are more flexible, and more thera-peutic than previously believed. Catherine Verfaillie has shown that adult stem cells are nearly as versatile as embryonic stem cells. Adult cells taken from the bone marrow of mice have developed into the cells of liver, lung, brain, and blood. They readily transformed these cells into liver cells but not so readily into heart cells.[22] The efficacy of adult stem cells circumvent ethi-cal problems with deriving stem cells from aborted fetuses and embryos, and it provides scientific advantages as well. Utilizing a patient's own adult stem cells would not run the risk of rejection, as would use of embryonic stem cells.[23] Also, proving to be less flexible may actually be advantageous for some purposes.

If adult stem cells have restricted instead of unlimited potential to de-velop into different tissues, that means the adult stem cells are farther along in their final stage of development.[24] Achieving the intended purpose of adult stem cells would require fewer interventions. As Maureen Condic explains, "if a patient with heart disease can be cured using adult cardiac stem cells, the fact that these 'heart restricted' stem cells do not generate kidneys is not a problem for the patient."[25]

5. Conclusion

In conclusion, embryonic stem cell research is morally justified, because bio-logical and cognitive developments are crucial factors for our moral delibera-tions. We cannot legitimately sacrifice other beings that deserve full moral consideration for the sake of transplant candidates.

Blastocysts, embryos, and fetuses do not deserve full moral considera-tion in virtue of their rudimentary biological level. Whether early human life forms deserve any moral status is an interesting issue. Like the issue of re-spect for the dead, debate over the moral status of early human life suggests that we should consider the moral value of rituals and other symbolic actions. Without developing a case for the symbolic value of early human life forms, it appears that they do not deserve much moral regard unless the intention is that they will become persons deserving of full moral consideration.

If adult stem cells prove equally therapeutic, there will be no scientific or moral justification for performing embryonic stem cell research, no matter how slight the moral status of blastocysts, embryos, and fetuses. In this case, embryonic stem cell research could only be morally justified if blastocysts, embryos, and fetuses have no moral status. Even then such research would be imprudent given the political issues involving early life forms. In this case, if we can avoid conflicts among right-to-life advocates, those depend-ing on scientific research, and parents' reproductive rights, especially women's, then we ought to avoid those conflicts. The problems are that adult stem cells have not been found in all tissues, and stem cell research is a new science. In the next chapter, I comment on a form of residue called the regulative principle that states we ought to avoid or eliminate conflict.

Part Three

A PHILOSOPHICAL RESPONSE

Ten

THE REGULATIVE PRINCIPLE

[E]ven though we should see how to lessen or eliminate certain conflicts, I do not think we have, or even could have, any real idea of how to
do this completely or in general. The present world and those worlds we
should think we could bring about are worlds of conflict.[1]

The previous chapters addressed several residue-producing conflicts with organ retrieval practices and proposals. Even when we respond with justification to these conflicts, our choices often result in considerable moral losses. In
response to these losses, scientists, healthcare providers, legal analysts, policy
makers, and ethics consultants have made or recommended adjustments to retrieve more organs and to protect other values as well. In this chapter, I link
the previous analysis with another alleged type of moral residue—reasons or
requirements to avoid conflicts or dilemmas.

1. Marcus's Regulative Principle

Recall that dilemmas involve situations where a person faces two moral requirements in some strong sense that she probably cannot both satisfy. By
contrast, in a conflict, a person faces a situation with two different values that
she probably cannot both realize, but one or neither of the values imposes a
requirement on the person. With conflicts, persons face incompatible moral recommendations, or the incompatibility of a requirement and a recommendation.

Ruth Charlotte Barcan Marcus claims we ought to adjust our lives and institutions in a way that minimizes dilemmas and conflicts—the regulative principle. The regulative principle is plausible assuming dilemmas necessitate
wrongdoing. We ought to avert, minimize, or cease wrongdoing. Not all dilemma defenders believe dilemmas make wrongdoing inevitable. Responding
to conflicts that are not dilemmas can also leave us with substantial losses. I
will evaluate the regulative principle as it applies to dilemmas that might make
wrongdoing inevitable and to non-dilemmatic conflicts. Although this analysis
does not cover all of the nuances associated with dilemmas, it does advance
our understanding of the regulative principle. I argue that the regulative principle is true for dilemmas as long as the non-moral reasons bearing on a case or
policy do not override the moral reasons for that case or policy, but that the
regulative principle is false for conflicts. Nevertheless we can agree with Marcus that we ought to avoid, eliminate, or minimize some conflicts and that we
ought to alleviate the moral losses that stem from conflicts. I also believe that

Marcus's comment that the regulative principle illustrates the dynamic character of the moral life has not received proper attention. With all of this in mind, I ultimately amend the regulative principle to say that our values guide our behavior and attitudes in the face of conflicts by giving us reason to make adjustments to avoid or alleviate moral losses.

Since Marcus does not clarify the meaning, application, or ramifications of the regulative principle, it helps to examine her words:

> Although dilemmas are not settled without residue, the recognition of their reality has a dynamic force. It motivates us to arrange our lives and institutions with a view to avoiding such conflicts. It is the underpinning for a second-order principle: that as rational agents with some control of our lives and institutions, we ought to conduct our lives and arrange our institutions to minimize predicaments of moral conflict.[2]

Notice that Marcus does not distinguish between dilemmas and conflicts, which she appears to regard as synonyms. Marcus's decision not to distinguish dilemmas from conflicts does not present an insurmountable obstacle to evaluating the regulative principle so long as we keep in mind the difference between dilemmas and conflicts discussed in the first chapter. Alternatively, a conflict may also involve disvalues, one of which a person will probably realize. Remember too that the implications of dilemmas are debatable. According to some philosophers, a person facing a dilemma is condemned to inevitable wrongdoing or something that is cause for guilt, regret, or remorse.

Other philosophers believe that a person facing a dilemma invariably does something that leaves residue, but the person does not necessarily do anything wrong or something about which the person should feel guilty. In this chapter, I only discuss the most controversial form of alleged dilemmas, a situation that makes wrongdoing inevitable, and a type of conflict that leaves us with residue.

To understand the regulative principle and its implications for ethics and medical ethics, we should understand that Marcus meant the regulative principle to solve a special problem within ethical theory. Marcus is a prominent logician who believes in dilemmas. Many philosophers believe that a commitment to the existence of dilemmas means that even the best possible moral theory will leave us with an inconsistent moral code, a code of values unable to guide our actions in all circumstances. Not surprisingly, then, Marcus attempts to show that a commitment to dilemmas does not mean we are left with an inconsistent moral code. That is, dilemmas do not show that even the best moral code will invariably leave us with conflicting directives. For example, it would be absurd for a moral code to tell us to proceed with embryonic stem cell research and not to proceed with embryonic stem cell research. Marcus claims that a moral code is consistent so long as the code might never yield conflicting directives; consistency does not mean that we will always be able to do what morality requires or recommends. This point is significant and deserves clarification.

To say that x is logically possible means that x is not contradictory; it does not mean that x is actually true. To say that a moral code may possibly yield only directives that can be satisfied means that we can imagine a world wherein that code never yields contradictory advice as to what we ought to do in real-life circumstances. The logical possibility of a consistent moral code does not mean that persons will never face contradictory moral directives in real-life situations. Consequently, if we feel trapped in a dilemma, it may not be that our moral code is defective in terms of its ability to guide our actions. It may mean that life has made impossible demands on us—what dilemma defenders have been telling us.

We may be disappointed with our moral code if its directives conflict in real life, even if the code is consistent in Marcus's technical sense. In articulating the regulative principle, Marcus wants to show that a moral code guides our actions even when dilemmas or conflicts indicate situations where our moral code fails to guide us. Marcus claims that a meta-principle directs us to avoid or eliminate conflicts or dilemmas. In this way, she defends the existence of dilemmas while preserving the view that morality is action guiding. Think about the importance of Marcus's view: if morality does not guide our actions, what is the purpose of morality? Perhaps surprisingly, the regulative principle has not received much attention from philosophers, but Marcus's view is helpful so I will first summarize how Mary Mothersill has criticized the regulative principle, and then present my views.

2. Mothersill on the Regulative Principle

Philosophers have not devoted much attention to the regulative principle. Terrance McConnell agrees that we should avoid conflicts but denies that the regulative principle provides any evidence that dilemmas exist.[3] Mary Mothersill claims that she does not know what Marcus means by saying we ought to arrange our institutions to avoid conflict. In her words it:

> sounds odd to ask someone to compare, for example, Columbia University with IBM with respect to their success in forestalling moral conflicts. Perhaps something like having a reasonable parental-leave policy that would not force employees to choose between their careers and child care would be counted.[4]

Mothersill claims that Kant's second formulation of the categorical imperative that states we ought to treat people as ends-in-themselves instead of as means to fulfill our desires justifies the parental-leave policy. We do not need to appeal to the regulative principle to clarify the morality of IBM's or Columbia's parental-leave policy. Although an interesting suggestion, I do not believe that Mothersill has succeeded in undermining the regulative principle.

Mothersill misses Marcus's point because she does not entertain the prospect of the employer having an opportunity to lose anything of moral value in granting a person a leave of absence. Mothersill claims that "the desire to manipulate and coerce other people proves a motive for devising situations that will be dilemmatic for them and that this is morally indefensible."[5] There may be a conflict between an employer and employees regarding parental leaves of absence, but that does not mean a moral value conflict is present. Corporations have treated their employees as less than fully human for the sake of profits and many corporations ought to implement an ethical parental-leave policy. Kant's second formulation of the categorical imperative and Marcus's regulative principle do not address the same ethical issues and would not always entail the same moral consequences. Avoiding conflict may mean showing respect for persons, but that will not always be the case. Also, the regulative principle addresses cases where respecting one person is incompatible with respecting another person. But Mothersill's disagreement with Marcus runs deep, so we must address her other concerns.

While Marcus believes that the contingencies of life make it so that our familiar moral principles make conflicting demands on us, Mothersill claims that we can describe every action in many ways. In addition, according to Mothersill, an action can fall under two or more descriptions that lead to conflicting advice. One description can forbid an action while another description prescribes that action. Apparently, accurate conflicting descriptions indicate a genuine conflict. I am not sure exactly what Mothersill means, but I do know that she thinks the regulative principle would amount to actions only satisfying a single description. That conclusion does not follow because a plurality of descriptions can offer consistent directives.

Finally, Mothersill believes that the directive that we ought to avoid conflict can be satisfied in undesirable ways. She says, "One way of avoiding moral conflict is to cut down on the number of one's obligations or to resolve to worry less about what precisely they are."[6] For example, by making fewer promises, we run less risk that we may have to break them for the sake of other values. Similarly, we could decide not to have children so that our parental requirements would never conflict with requirements to spouses, family members, strangers, or employers. The surest way to avoid conflict would be for no one to have children and for us to allow the human species to become extinct!

These absurd consequences could follow from Marcus's regulative principle only if it were the only moral principle she endorsed. Marcus does not intend the regulative principle as a supreme principle for us to follow under all circumstances. I agree with Mothersill that the regulative principle needs to be qualified, but Mothersill's last objection misses the spirit of Marcus's point. Her recommendation is to avoid conflict as much as possible while pursuing our values, not to avoid conflict at all costs.

3. The Regulative Principle and Dilemmas

It may appear obviously true that we ought to avoid or eliminate dilemmas. After all, although non-dilemmatic conflicts can generate losses and residue, only a designated conception of dilemmas, what I will call the narrow sense, threatens persons with inevitable wrongdoing. It appears true that we ought to avoid wrongdoing. To accept the existence of dilemmas in the narrow sense and reject the regulative principle suggests that wrongdoing is permissible in some cases, perhaps even required all things considered in some cases. To call an action or omission wrong all things considered means that the action or omission is not morally permissible. Accepting the existence of dilemmas while rejecting the regulative principle on moral grounds appears to violate our linguistic conventions by leading us into a contradiction. How, then, can we sensibly deny the regulative principle if we also believe in dilemmas in the narrow sense?

One tempting strategy to show that accepting the narrow conception of dilemmas and rejecting the regulative principle does not lead to a contradiction would be to say that wrongdoing can be instrumental or necessary to produce a greater good or to avoid an even greater wrong. For this view, a wrong action might be permissible. According to this strategy, for example, Sophie does wrong by choosing her daughter to die in order to prevent the Nazis from killing both children, but we still consider her choice permissible. On a lesser scale than Sophie's choice, transplant teams sometimes lie to family members of a transplant candidate about why they rejected a relative as a candidate for live-kidney donation. If the relative who is a potential donor indicated that he did not want to donate, transplant teams will sometimes lie by saying that the person was medically unsuitable to be a donor. In such a case, one might say that the wrong of telling the lie is justified by the good of sparing the reluctant relative from shame and mistreatment from his relatives.

The problem with this strategy of reconciling dilemmas in the narrow sense with a rejection of the regulative principle is that it misrepresents all-things-considered moral judgments. If, say, lying is justified in a case, then we must accept that lying is morally permissible for that case. We can and should acknowledge that even if lying in such cases is morally permissible, telling the lie is morally undesirable in that case as well. This last point might tempt people to think that even morally permissible decisions can be wrong. As the arguments in the first chapter showed, we can acknowledge that permissible decisions can include moral losses and leave us with residue without concluding that the decisions are wrong. We have no conceptual need to engage in double-speak about how an action can be wrong all things considered but permissible. For these reasons, I think defenders of dilemmas must accept the regulative principle so long as we think of dilemmas as making wrongdoing inevitable, and so long as we assume that non-moral reasons do not override the moral reasons bearing on the case.

It might be that non-moral reasons can override moral reasons in some cases. For example, it might be true that moral considerations indicate that we ought to presume individuals wish to donate their organs or that we ought to routinely retrieve organs as needed. There might be political and legal reasons for not implementing such policies. For these cases, saying dilemmas exist, but that we should not avoid or eliminate all of these dilemmas once we consider all of the non-moral reasons, is coherent. Even if we are considering a narrow conception of dilemma, the regulative principle will not necessarily be true for all cases when we consider non-moral considerations. I stated at the beginning of this book that I am interested in the moral dimensions of residue-producing conflicts. As long as we restrict our discussion to moral reasons, Marcus is correct in thinking that we will always have moral reasons to avoid or eliminate dilemmas in the narrow sense.

Another problem for the regulative principle arises with the definition of dilemma as a situation that makes wrongdoing inevitable. As we learned in chapter one, this conception of dilemma is the most controversial form of dilemma, and many philosophers do not believe such dilemmas exist. If dilemmas that make wrongdoing inevitable do not exist, the regulative principle is true only in theory for dilemmas; it can have no practical application. Even if these dilemmas exist, if they rarely occur, the regulative principle will have severely limited application. What we need is to examine the application of the regulative principle to types of conflicts that are commonplace.

For those who believe dilemmas exist, but that they do not entail inevitable wrongdoing, my analysis of the regulative principle as applied to conflicts is relevant. As was demonstrated in chapter one, the difference between some conceptions of dilemmas and conflicts is largely semantic. What I conclude about the regulative principle as applied to residue-producing conflicts might also hold true for some conceptions of a dilemma, depending on the sort of distinctions we make between conflicts and dilemmas. I argue that the regulative principle cannot be true for conflicts even when we restrict our judgments to moral considerations. After clarifying the meaning of the regulative principle for conflicts, I argue that we should not avoid or eliminate some conflicts all things considered. Yet, residue-producing conflicts are obviously relevant to our future moral planning, and that planning must include avoiding and eliminating some conflicts.

4. The Regulative Principle and Conflicts

The intuitive idea behind the regulative principle for conflicts is that, all other things remaining equal, the realization of two values is better than the realization of only one value and the occurrence of two disvalues is worse than the occurrence of only one disvalue. We might render a first pass at developing an interpretation of the regulative principle regarding conflicting values in the following way. If we must choose between circumstance $c1$ in which two values are satisfied and $c2$ in which one of those two values is violated or unrealized, we should attempt to realize $c1$ in favor of $c2$ all other things being equal. Unless our efforts make it possible to realize both values, value conflicts entail we must sacrifice one value, or realize one disvalue. The point of the regulative principle is that we ought to try to avoid or eliminate conflicts for the sake of bringing more value into our lives and eliminating as much disvalue as possible.

The regulative principle circumvents the problem of weighing values to resolve a conflict. If it turns out that we can satisfy two values that were on a collision course or avoid the realization of a disvalue, we do not have to worry with weighing the values so that we can act in accordance with the value with the greatest weight. Instead, our challenge becomes one of making institutional, psychological, political, scientific, or conceptual adjustments to avoid or eliminate the conflict. The only priority ranking is in the claim that making adjustments so that we can realize both values in a conflict is better than only realizing one of those values, and avoiding two disvalues is better than having to tolerate one disvalue. That said, I want to show that several examples from organ retrieval and transplantation lend plausibility to the regulative principle when applied to conflicts. I then show that, despite that initial plausibility, the regulative principle cannot be true for all conflicts all things considered.

Suppose two persons suffer from severe liver damage. A transplant surgeon must decide which one will be the beneficiary of a donated liver. Suppose that each of the patients would benefit from this transplant. If transplant surgeons could find a way to benefit both patients, it would be preferable to help both of them instead of just one, assuming no other relevant factors.

Fortunately, recent technological advances make possible the division of donor livers into two separate transplantable lobes offering the opportunity to save both of the liver transplant candidates. Before the development of this procedure, members of the transplant community often faced the terrible choice of deciding which of two or more persons should receive an available liver for transplantation. Transplant technology such as that allowing for the division of livers into separate transplantable lobes reflects the spirit of the regulative principle; find a way to avoid or alleviate conflicts.

Adjustments to avoid moral conflicts are not restricted to technological advancements. Take another example from the common apparent conflict between respecting the prior wishes of decedents to donate their organs and their families' opposition to having their organs taken. To avoid this conflict, the transplant community encourages familial discussion of donation in the hope that donors and their families can reach agreement, or that their families will honor their relative's former wishes if the occasion arises. Members of transplant teams know to approach families with sensitivity to avoid trampling upon families' moral and aesthetic sensibilities. In this way, we increase the chances that we respect the former wishes of the dead without violating the family members' values or exacerbating their grief. Good communication among family members also meets the obvious goal of extending transplant candidates' lives.

These considerations also show that encouraging families to discuss donation and training members of transplant teams to approach families with sensitivity are like the technological advancement of dividing livers in that they are strategies for arranging our lives to avoid conflicts, thereby bringing more value into the world. Avoiding conflicts is not the only or primary reason to encourage open discussion among family members regarding organ donation, but it provides one reason, and it helps us to appreciate the spirit of the regulative principle. We need not accept that we should avoid or eliminate all value conflicts all morally relevant factors considered.

Given the complexities of life, we have good reason to tolerate some conflicts for a while, because avoiding or eliminating conflicts can have undesirable moral consequences. Many technological developments generate conflicts while producing much good. A kidney transplant, for example, can relieve a patient from the pain and dehumanization of hemodialysis. Kidney transplants overcome the conflict patients have to face when having to choose between either avoiding suffering by refusing dialysis and dying, or living with the discomfort and anguish of hemodialysis. Kidney transplants also create a conflict between the value of extending a patient's life and the value of being free from the pain of transplantation and the side effects of immunosuppressive treatment.

In many cases, the value of extending life through hemodialysis or a transplant outweighs the dehumanization of hemodialysis or post-transplant suffering. A kidney transplant often improves the quality of life of patients who were receiving hemodialysis. The acknowledgment of conflicts created by the development of kidney transplantation does not mean that surgeons should never have developed kidney transplants. This is Mothersill's point, albeit overstated by suggesting that the regulative principle is superfluous.

Consider another case. Receiving a kidney from a living relative often proves to be better for a transplant recipient than receiving a transplant from a non-related cadaver.[7] Unfortunately, conflicts sometimes arise because the optimal health of the patient requires the living relative to make a sacrifice that the relative does not wish to make. This does not mean they should never have developed living-donor kidney transplants.

The aforementioned reflections show moral grounds for avoiding some conflicts and that we ought to perform some actions even though they lead to conflicts. Even if all of the morally relevant factors in a case indicate that we ought to tolerate a conflict for the sake of a good or combination of goods, we can still have reason to alleviate the fallout of the conflict. So, even if we must accept occasional conflicts between living kidney donors and their relatives who could benefit from their donation, we can try to alleviate the conflict by developing safer surgical methods and better immunosuppressive drugs to alleviate donors' risks and fears. By accounting for these straightforward observations, we can attain Marcus's goal of showing that morality is action guiding without defending the view that we ought to avoid or eliminate all conflicts. Still, we should recognize a deeper point about the regulative principle.

5. Preventive Medicine

Recall that Marcus mentions the dynamic character of the moral life when she introduces the regulative principle. If critics of the regulative principle had emphasized Marcus's interest in the dynamic character of the moral life, instead of emphasizing her claim that we ought to avoid or eliminate conflicts, I think many more philosophers would appreciate the regulative principle. What we need to say is that residue-producing conflicts provide some reason to avoid or eliminate conflicts and to alleviate the losses from making a choice between conflicting values, or to acknowledge the fallout. In turn, a choice between conflicting values changes the world in some way that both provides new opportunities to realize values and leads to more residue-producing conflicts. The new residue-producing conflicts, then, present us with new choices and new reasons to exercise choice. I think Marcus has this dynamic feature of the moral life in mind when she introduces the regulative principle. The dynamism of the moral life becomes even more interesting with issues such as organ retrieval strategies because of the many conceptual, technological, psychological, legal, and social adjustments that we have and can make in the attempt to make the world a better place. Although knowing which adjustments we should make can be difficult, an obvious application of the regulative principle to organ retrieval has received surprisingly little attention.

Virtually all of the commentators on the ethics of organ retrieval and transplantation omit to discuss the prevention of organ failure. This omission is surprising since it would be obviously good if few people needed a transplant. If few people needed a transplant, we could avoid many residue-producing conflicts. One reason commentators do not discuss preventive measures is that many of the reasons for organ failure are unknown or difficult to prevent. But we do know some diseases that lead to organ failure are preventable. Factors leading to the development of coronary artery disease are a high-fat diet, smoking, and a sedentary lifestyle. Alcohol abuse can lead to cirrhosis and, in severe cases, cardiomyopathy, and obesity is a significant factor in diabetes that often results in kidney failure. Most of us know that eating well and exercising can reduce the risk of many of the diseases that lead to or contribute to organ failure. We can do a better job of promoting health as individuals, as societies, and as a global community.

Although American society does a good job of informing people about the health benefits of eating well and exercising, we could do better. We could, for instance, develop good tasting, healthful fast food. We could also do a much better job of discouraging persons from abusing alcohol. I find it strange and morally dubious that clinicians and medical ethicists encourage the redefinition of death and the development of xenotransplantation but say nothing or virtually nothing about preventive measures or measures to encourage healthier lifestyles in response to premature organ failure. That commentators discuss many approaches to retrieve more organs more often than they discuss preventive measures reflects research trends, commentators' biases, and the dominant rhetoric of organ retrieval.

Most commentators describe the disparity between those who could benefit from a transplant and the number of available organs as an organ shortage. This may appear like common sense, but we should stop and ask why clinicians and medical ethicists have not described the problem as a surplus of people suffering from congenital or premature organ failure. Describing the disparity as an organ shortage or as a surplus of people suffering from organ failure appears to have the same meaning and yield the same practical consequences, but organ transplant discussion and research efforts suggest otherwise. Whether as a symptom, causal contributor, or both, the rhetoric of organ retrieval fits the aggressive measures taken or recommended to retrieve more organs. Awareness of our value-laden language affords us the opportunity to acknowledge and, perhaps, transcend our prejudices, and expand our opportunities to address the need for organ transplantation as a problem of premature or congenital organ failure.

6. Conclusion

The regulative principle is true for the narrow conception of dilemma so long as we restrict our analysis to moral reasons. The problem is that the narrow conception of dilemma is the most controversial form of dilemma. Many philosophers do not believe such dilemmas exist. Even if these dilemmas exist, unless there are many, the regulative principle will not guide our actions often. For non-dilemmatic residue-producing conflicts, the regulative principle is not true for many cases. Yet, Marcus has done well to remind us that making the world a better place often includes avoiding or minimizing conflicts.

The organ retrieval and transplant community should emphasize ways to prevent organ failure. Although I reject a literal interpretation of the regulative principle for many conflicts, I retain its spirit by revising it to account for two facts: we ought not avoid or eliminate all conflicts, and we ought to mitigate the moral losses resulting from our choices. An emended version of the regulative principle should say that our values give us reason to make adjustments to avoid or eliminate conflicts or to alleviate the moral fallout resulting from conflicts; adjustments may be conceptual, psychological, legal, scientific, medical, institutional, or technological.

It will not always be possible to make an adjustment to alleviate the fallout of conflicting values related to organ retrieval. This inability creates a problem for Marcus's attempt to preserve the action-guiding nature of morality that the acknowledgment of dilemmas superficially undermines. As the dilemma literature shows, dilemmas and conflicts affect our emotional lives. The desire to retain the action-guiding nature of morality while also recognizing the emotional impact of moral conflicts leads Patricia Greenspan to say that emotional responses indicate the motivational force of moral language.[8]

I find it more plausible to say that morality is response guiding instead of merely action guiding; emotional responses are among the types of responses that warrant moral evaluation. Regarding morality as response guiding easily accommodates the spirit of the regulative principle by acknowledging the dynamic nature of the moral life and the view that morality is guiding.

Even in cases where we cannot prevent a conflict or alleviate a moral loss resulting from a conflicting choice, we can preserve the view of morality as guiding by acknowledging psychological responses. Regarding morality as response guiding is consistent with Michael Stocker's and Elizabeth Anderson's call to find ways to reconcile ethical views that emphasize a person's character with ethical views that emphasize the importance of correct action independent of a person's character.[9]

The crucial question for our purposes is what sorts of adjustments we should make, especially when some of our choices involve incommensurable values and when concepts such as hope, luck, and commitment to a project comprise much of the character of moral life. In the next chapter, I sketch a normative and meta-analysis of decision-making in light of these challenges.

Eleven

CONSTRUCTIVE PLURALISM

The previous chapters demonstrated and anticipated the morality of adopting different organ retrieval strategies. I indicated my support for the sale of organs retrieved after the seller's death, embryonic and adult stem cell research, and keeping the Dead Donor Rule. I also expressed opposition to routine retrieval, adopting a higher brain definition of death, retrieving organs from living sellers, and the xenotransplantation of whole organs. I have not found compelling reason to reject or support presumed consent or the cardiopulmonary definition of death. Room for reasonable disagreement on many of these issues remains, because identifying all of the relevant values is difficult, and comparing the benefits and burdens of adopting strategies with sufficient precision is often challenging or unlikely. In this chapter, I argue that we can make reasonable and justifiable decisions regarding organ retrieval policy even if incommensurable choices are commonplace.

1. Routine Retrieval, Presumed Consent, and Familial Consent

In chapter three, I explored whether we can wrong the dead and whether routine retrieval, presumed consent, and familial consent can violate the former wishes of the dead. Like many people, I believe we ought to respect the dead and that routine retrieval, presumed consent, and familial consent can violate respect for the dead. Yet a compelling reason for respecting the dead remains elusive. With this challenge in mind, can we assert with confidence that respect for the dead takes priority over the needs of the living? Even if we determine that we can wrong the dead by practicing routine retrieval, presumed consent, or familial consent, how can we gain a good sense of the extent or severity of the wrong?

Another problem with resolving the apparent conflict between respecting the dead and helping more transplant candidates involves evaluating the moral import of living persons' reactions to strategies. If we routinely retrieve organs or implement a policy of presumed consent, how could we measure the disappointment of living individuals opposed to these policies? How would people react if we abolished the practice of familial consent? Social scientists can help us determine the public's attitudes, but social science cannot show us how we ought to evaluate a policy. After all, we still must address whether we should attempt to shape public opinions to tolerate or embrace routine retrieval or presumed consent, or reject familial consent. In the final analysis, I do not see how we are supposed to compare the value of respecting the former wishes of the dead with the value of extending life for transplant candidates with anything other than vague, albeit powerful, intuitions.

2. The Definition of Death

When selecting a definition of death, three conspicuous moral issues emerge. We must consider the impact of each definition on retrieving organs. The definition must be credible in that it accurately captures the meaning of death lest we sacrifice our integrity. We must also carefully weigh the value of treating with respect prospective organ donors or sellers who are near death.

All other things being equal, the higher brain definition of death would lead to the retrieval of more organs. Given that many people, including many healthcare professionals, do not believe whole brain death constitutes death, we can be sure that even fewer people would accept the higher brain definition. The higher brain definition of death leads us to disrespect those barely alive by treating them as if they are dead and risks diminishing the integrity of those who propagate a definition of death they do not sincerely believe.

The cardiopulmonary definition declares death later than do the higher brain and whole brain definitions. Consequently, unless we follow Robert Truog's suggestion to retrieve organs from those barely alive, or we further develop organ retrieval from non-heart-beating cadavers, implementing this definition will result in fewer transplantable organs. If we want to follow Truog's suggestion, we would have to compare the value of extending life for transplant candidates with the moral and social problem of actively killing those barely alive. Those who find Truog's suggestion distasteful and morally dubious or outrageous may believe the whole brain definition remains our best option. But the whole brain definition may not lead to the retrieval of as many organs.

We have difficult comparisons to make regarding the truth about defining death, the treatment of those barely alive, and the value of retrieving more organs. I reject the higher brain definition because it does not accurately reflect ordinary discourse, and I do not think that we should take organs from persons in a persistent vegetative state even if their family members would consent. We should not abandon the Dead Donor Rule either. But we should understand that regardless of our support or rejection of some policies, we have more vague intuitions or debatable principles regarding value comparisons between helping transplant candidates and respecting those barely alive.

3. Selling Organs

I have argued that retrieving organs from living individuals willing to sell organs disrespects persons but that retrieving organs from sellers after they die is morally permissible.

While we have plausible reasons to prohibit the retrieval of organs from living sellers, such a prohibition risks allowing more transplant candidates to die all other things being equal. How are we supposed to compare the value of respecting persons' bodies against the value of preventing the premature deaths of those who will die while waiting for a transplant? The answer is impossible to specify precisely, in part, because we do not know how many transplant candidates would benefit from live-organ sales. Doubtless, the number of lives saved would partially depend upon the price given for the organs. Yet, guidelines do not precisely show how the commodification of our organs diminishes respect for persons.

4. Xenotransplants

With xenotransplantation, we must assess the value of the lives of transplant candidates in comparison to the disvalue of killing pigs and of risking the spread of disease to transplant candidates and to third parties. To make justified evaluations we must have some idea of how many pigs' lives would be lost and how many xenotransplant recipients would have their lives extended at quantitatively and qualitatively meaningful levels. Another obstacle is that experts disagree over the risks to third parties, and, frankly, their opinion rests on many hunches, fears, and hopes. Proceeding cautiously through clinical trials removes some of the guesswork from the equation, but not all of it. With so much uncertainty, it will be difficult to make a compelling case for any final evaluation of xenotransplantation. But we should be reluctant to accept more risky strategies such as the xenotransplantation of whole organs.

5. Stem Cell Research

Embryonic stem cell research is justified because transplant candidates are worth more than embryos and fetuses all other things remaining equal. I realize that many persons passionately feel otherwise. Although I disagree with them, their reactions to policies are morally relevant.

The pro-life movement demonstrates that many persons are outraged over the termination of nascent human life forms. How much weight should we give to negative emotional responses to research on embryonic stem cells and other such practices? How are we supposed to compare the grief of right-to-life advocates with that of persons whose loved ones died while waiting for transplants? We cannot provide precise answers, but I believe that the preponderance of the moral considerations indicates that we ought to vigorously pursue stem cell research. Adult stem cells avoid moral and political conflicts over the moral status of embryos and fetuses and have the potential for reducing premature organ failure. Embryonic stem cell research might prove the most therapeutic in virtue of greater versatility.

6. Reasonable Decisions Despite Incommensurability

In the light of the limitations of our moral intuitions, the indeterminacy of conventional medical ethics, and the incommensurability of values, I suggest we view organ retrieval strategies as a constructive process providing reasons and requirements to make a series of adjustments to residue-producing conflicts. Despite the problem of incommensurability, we can rationally respond to these conflicts by regarding organ retrieval as a project involving many strategies, each of which requires a commitment to realize values and a willingness to make adjustments for moral losses. Although we cannot always alleviate losses, this analysis shows that morality can be action guiding without suggesting we should always or most often expect there to be a single justified or best set of actions or strategies, even when our options are not morally equal. I also discuss a tension between regarding our organ retrieval strategies as a large project consisting of incommensurable values and our inclination to find the best answer to the question, what practices should we adopt to address the problem of premature or congenital organ failure?

The approach I take to responding to moral conflicts is common in many respects but unconventional in the way a series of actions and strategies shape decisions and the way we view our moral lives. I have not found many likeminded ethical theorists or applied ethicists, but Terrance McConnell's position on responding to incommensurable conflicts resonates with my view. He may not agree with my approach, but his exposition helps clarify what I mean by constructive pluralism.

McConnell develops his insights on rational decision-making when a person faces incommensurable alternatives in response to Gerald Paske's essay on dilemmas that require us to choose between incommensurable values. Paske argues that incommensurable values help explain the intractability of dilemmas.[1] McConnell, on the other hand, offers moral guidance even in the context of choosing between incommensurable values.

McConnell argues that, even when faced with conflicts involving incommensurable values, reason does not leave us with merely a flip of a coin. He links decisions involving value conflicts to a broader context involving the "morally best scenario of actions."[2] He is suggesting that even if a single initial response to a choice between incommensurable values is arbitrary, whatever decision a person makes constitutes the first step in a series of actions aiming to achieve a justifiable overall balance of values. By shifting our emphasis from finding unique correct responses involving moral choice to a broader context including a series of actions, much of the moral life looks like a creative endeavor, a constructive process. This process includes adjustments to build upon the value of a selected path, to prevent conflicts, and to alleviate the fallout resulting from our choices, even good choices.

Suppose, for example, that we do not know whether a world in which we vigorously pursue the development of xenotransplantation is better than, worse than, or morally equal to a world in which we do not pursue xenotransplantation. Still, we would know that a world in which we carefully conduct clinical trials related to xenotransplantation and develop better methods to eradicate the transmission of viruses and bacteria is better than a world in which we rush to perform xenotransplantation and make no serious efforts to prevent the transmission of harmful microorganisms.

This evaluation is true whether we support the xenotransplantation of whole organs or whether embarking on xenotransplantation involves making some choices between incommensurable values. The commensurability of all evaluations related to whether we should proceed with xenotransplantation is not necessary to make other commensurable choices related to xenotransplantation. Put another way, even if we face incommensurable options or think that we might face incommensurable choices after much deliberation, we can still justifiably rule out some series of options on moral grounds.

Consider also that we decide not to implement the higher brain definition of death on the basis that it does not adequately reflect what we mean by "death." If implementing the higher brain definition is morally impermissible, then it follows that it would be morally impermissible to retrieve organs from persons in a permanent vegetative state. If all other retrieval strategies remained the same as what we presently have in the United States, we would retrieve fewer organs than if we implemented the higher brain definition and persons in a persistent vegetative state became sources of organs. In making the decision not to implement the higher brain definition, we recognize that more transplant candidates will die while waiting for transplants unless we make other adjustments in current organ retrieval strategies.

For example, we could adopt a policy like the Pittsburgh protocol where we retrieve organs from non-heart-beating cadavers. Alternatively, we could do as Truog suggests; abandon the Dead Donor rule and retrieve organs from persons who are barely alive. Alternatively, we could find some other way to retrieve more organs. Such suggestions arise due to needed adjustments in response to a prior decision on the definition of death. The point is that we must evaluate our decision on the higher brain definition in the context of decisions on many related issues.

Regardless whether values are commensurable, we must assess our actions in terms of a series of actions that will include sets of strategies. In the case of incommensurable alternatives, to make a reasonable decision that is not arbitrary or akin to flipping a coin, we only have to have good grounds for thinking that *one series of actions* is better than, less than, or equal to an *alternative series of actions*. For this reason, the value of *single actions* may be incommensurable while a series of actions that includes one or more incommensurable options may be commensurable with alternative series of actions. That is, individual choices can be incommensurable while a series of actions are commensurable. For example, suppose we do not know whether the moral status of adult pigs is greater than, less than, or equal to the moral status of early human life forms such as blastocysts, embryos, and fetuses in early stages. Still, we might know that embryonic and adult stem cell research is justified and that successful stem cell research is better than unsuccessful xenotransplant research.

Failure to recognize valuations such as these has led some philosophers to overestimate the problems associated with widespread incommensurability. Recall that the worry is that incommensurable choices undermine the rationality of our decision-making. Recognition of the need to think about moral decision-making in terms of a series of actions leaves us with the challenge of comparing the value of different series of actions, or, let us say, different sets of actions. So, we should consider the value of different series of actions related to organ retrieval strategies. Considering sets of strategies provides an opportunity to clarify the importance of the distinction between evaluating individual options and evaluating different series of actions.

7. Sets of Strategies

Some may be tempted to think that the way to evaluate a set of organ retrieval strategies is to evaluate each strategy individually and then conclude that the conjunction of individually justifiable strategies constitutes the best set. We could try to independently decide whether to adopt routine retrieval or presumed consent, a definition of death, an aggressive approach to xenotransplantation and stem cell research programs, and financial incentives for organs. After deciding upon each issue, we could combine them to have a justified or optimal set of policies. The value of a set of strategies would presumably be equal to the value of the sum of the individual strategies. But this cannot be the case.

Whenever multiple strategies affect a goal such as retrieving, repairing, or creating more transplantable organs, the overall value of one strategy can partly depend upon the overall value of other strategies. If, for example, financial incentives would lead to a sufficient number of persons selling their organs, the development of xenotransplantation would be superfluous. If organ sales failed to significantly increase the supply of organs and stem cell researchers encountered unexpected obstacles, then we would have greater reason to implement some other strategy such as presumed consent.

Having good reasons not to implement more risky strategies provides incentive to embark on measures that are more benign. Similarly, if the benign measures are ineffective, we have more reason to take greater risks. Such adjustments characterize the development of organ retrieval practices and proposals. Because voluntary donation and the adoption of the whole brain definition of death have not yielded sufficient numbers of transplantable organs, strategies such as xenotransplantation and stem cell research are more enticing.

Implementing a set of strategies will depend, in part, on weighing values we regard as commensurable. For example, a reasonable person could object to xenotransplants, routine retrieval, and the selling of organs on deontological grounds. It could be said that pigs, the dead, and living persons' bodies ought to be treated with respect and that this means we ought not implement xenotransplant programs, routine retrieval, presumed consent, or the retrieval of organs or lobes of organs from living sellers. We could plausibly say that even if the current United States system of altruistic donation, the definition of death, and the present status of stem cell research fail to allow us to retrieve, repair, or create sufficient organs, we cannot justify some policies.

The totality of organ retrieval strategies needs evaluation. This conclusion is not surprising but each strategy is a project that can develop in many ways, thereby yielding an unwieldy number of organ retrieval possibilities. We need to narrow down our options.

It may be true that some strategies can never, or in few circumstances, be justified. The deontologist in the above example would still have moral reasons to find other ways to assist transplant candidates, such as developing transplant science so that we can expand donor criteria, improving education about donation and transplantation, developing artificial organs, and so forth. To abandon one strategy for retrieving organs on moral grounds gives us moral reason to find some other way to help transplant candidates to avoid the loss of qualitatively meaningful lives. We must confront the challenge of comparing and prioritizing many alternative sets of policies.

Consider four representative partial sets for illustrative purposes: (1) an ambitious set, (2) a conservative set, (3) the current set of strategies in the United States, and (4) my recommended set. These four sets are not an exhaustive list. For example, I have not addressed the retrieval of organs from anencephalic infants and the development of artificial organs. Many more combinations of strategies exist. Each set requires continuous effort to realize values, avoid disvalues, and alleviate moral losses. The emphasis on continuous efforts and decisions on different strategies illustrates the importance of a series of actions for thinking about moral decision-making.

Admittedly, sincere, reasonable thinkers might raise plausible objections to any one of these sets of strategies. My purpose is to indicate that the problem of incommensurability limits us when we attempt to discover the best set. But we can compare and rationally rank some sets.

Set 1: We embrace a higher brain definition of death and we routinely retrieve organs. We also vigorously pursue the development of xenotransplants and embryonic and adult stem cell research. In the United

States, this would mean that the president would need to revise current rules. Since we routinely retrieve organs, we do not need presumed consent and selling organs to increase the organ supply. We also reject the Dead Donor Rule.

Set 2: In this scenario, we retain the whole brain definition of death, and we pursue xenotransplantation and adult stem cell research and embryonic stem cell research with existing embryonic lines. We keep the altruistic tradition of organ donation, instead of allowing persons to sell their organs. We continue to gain donor or familial consent before retrieving organs.

Set 3: We retain the whole brain definition of death, but adopt a policy of presumed consent. Since many people opt out of the process, we allow individuals to sell their organs that transplant teams retrieve after they die. We do not vigorously pursue xenotransplantation or stem cell research.

Set 4: We retain the whole brain definition of death, and we limit xenotransplantation to tissues and cells. We aggressively pursue embryonic and adult stem cell research and permit the sale of organs that they retrieve once the seller dies. We gain consent before retrieving organs from those who decide not to sell their organs. Finally, major preventive medicine programs are developed.

Set one, representing an ambitious set of strategies, would extend the lives of more people as effectively as any conjunction of strategies, but runs the risk of over-determining an adequate supply of organs. If we implemented routine retrieval, why would we need to develop xenotransplants? Conversely, if xenotransplantation proves to be as promising as some predict, why would we need to routinely take organs? One rationale for this set of strategies is that if one strategy proves less than completely successful, another strategy will allow for the retrieval of a sufficient number of organs. For example, if citizens revolted against the implementation of routine retrieval, xenotransplantation or stem cell research might meet the goals of transplantation.

Although resulting in retrieving the most organs, set one consists of the most controversial approaches to organ retrieval. Some countries might be willing to accept set one, but Americans may not be ready to accept these policies, especially the routine retrieval of organs.

Given the complex and largely unexplored notion of the dead having moral status, it would be imprudent to permit routine retrieval. Some may be tempted to abandon routine retrieval and retain the rest of the strategies in set one. If we accept Ray G. Frey's premise that moral worth is a function of the

ability to experience and create value, then we will have a difficult time justifying xenotransplantation as morally permissible while routine retrieval is not.
In contrast to living pigs, corpses have no experiences at all. In addition,
transplant recipients and third parties might contract diseases.

Set 2 contains the conjunction of policies that the United States presently
implements. This set does not generate much social discord, but as the organ
retrieval and transplant community reminds us, this set of policies allows
many persons to die while waiting for a transplant. No matter our moral perspective, we cannot deny that losing thousands of lives each year constitutes a
substantial loss. As transplantation medicine develops, more individuals can
benefit from transplantation; thus, transplant waiting lists will increase. In the
future, even more individuals will die from organ failure, unless future efforts
prove more helpful than do present efforts. Apparently, the death of those
waiting for a transplant does not bother many of us. Otherwise, more of us
would donate or find another way to help.

Overall, set 3 constitutes a conservative program. This set would likely
receive criticism for being too conservative, especially for not vigorously pursuing xenotransplantation and stem cell research. The decision to curb stem
cell research would probably have widespread implications for organ transplantation and other medical issues as well. This set would undermine our opportunities to have a sufficient number of available transplantable organs.
Anyone advocating this set would have moral reason to help transplant candidates in other ways. These advocates could limit the number of transplant
candidates by embarking on an ambitious preventive medicine campaign. If
successful, we could significantly decrease the number of individuals needing
an organ transplant in the future. Advocates of this set would have a lot of explaining to do as to why they are not doing more to help those with immediate
needs. Although implementing successful preventive medicine programs can
circumvent the need for many future organ transplants, the obstruction of
medical progress would be serious and unjustifiable.

Acting in accordance with my suggestions in set four would not allow
for the retrieval of as many organs as set 1 would yield. Regrettably, in the
short term, these procedures would result in the death of more transplant candidates. Yet, we must consider other values in times of conflicts. Protecting
values such as respect for persons, honesty in our treatment of the dead and
those near death, and protection of communities' health, imply that we should
not embark on the quest for organs with untempered zeal.

Since I also want to save as many transplant candidates as possible while
protecting other values, I must address residual reasons to solve the problem
of dying patients. For the long-term, I suggest that we devote substantial resources into preventive medicine.

Before undertaking to evaluate the sets of strategies, we should understand that each set contains incommensurable choices, and choosing among

some of the sets involves incommensurable choices. We do not know how to *precisely* compare the instrumental value of adult stem cell research with the instrumental value of xenotransplantation. Nor do I think a compelling argument exists that clarifies how to accurately compare the moral status of adult pigs or seriously compromised adult human beings with the value of early human life forms such as blastocysts, embryos, and fetuses. Although precise evaluations are not necessary for commensurability, imprecision can lead to incommensurable options.

Increasing the number of possible combinations of strategies considered by informed individuals and groups will increase the difficulty in finding agreement about which set of policies is best. Many medical ethicists write as if we can expect to find a single correct answer if we think well enough about the moral and empirical details of each strategy. I agree that we should continue to debate the moral and empirical issues, but I do not expect scholars individually or collectively to discover a best answer to the question, what strategies should we employ to help those with failing organs?

Despite these elements of incommensurability, we can make reasonable and justifiable decisions that are not arbitrary. We know that given adequate resources, good efforts to develop adult stem cell research are better than weak efforts to develop adult stem cell research. Since successful adult stem cell use does not destroy life as does xenotransplantation and some forms of embryonic stem cell research, we know that successful adult stem cell use is morally better than successful xenotransplantation and some forms of embryonic stem cell research, assuming adult stem cell therapy will be effective.

Shifting our emphasis from an individual choice between incommensurable options to a series of actions whereby we act in accordance with values and minimize moral losses shows how reasonable decisions can co-exist with widespread incommensurability. Even if many of our options are incommensurable, there can be enough commensurability to justify preferring some options to others. Each set implies that organ retrieval strategies require continuous effort.

Even widespread incommensurability does not undermine our ability to make intelligent choices. True, terms such as "widespread," "successful," "intelligent," and "reasonable" are vague, but we can still make good choices in cases of incommensurability. As long as we can make some accurate comparisons, we do not need a vast majority of our choices to be commensurable to lead qualitatively meaningful lives. What we need is the will to realize values and minimize losses through various adjustments.

A problem has been the assumption of a sharp division between incommensurable choices and commensurable choices. Given the arguments over moral status, uncertainties with successfully developing different research programs, imprecise moral intuitions, different personal and cultural proclivities, and the continuous adjustments that have been highlighted in previous chapters, we should expect nothing less than a complex mix of commensurable and incommensurable options. Such is the variegated landscape of moral choices.

The literature on organ retrieval reveals vigorous disagreement among advocates and critics over the ethics of individual organ retrieval strategies. Such disagreement does not show that the commentators have moral or rational flaws. In a world where some values are in dispute, where recognized values conflict and create moral losses no matter what we do, where some values are incommensurable, and where morally relevant outcomes depend upon present and future conceptual, political, institutional, scientific, legal, and psychological adjustments, we should expect uncertainty and disagreement. This need not make us pessimistic about whether we can make justified choices. Although not all organ retrieval strategies can be justified, we can select among a range of plausible sets of strategies and make adjustments along the way to avoid some conflicts and to alleviate our losses. Organ retrieval also demonstrates the totality of adjustments available to us, to think of applied ethics in terms of a series of actions, and to see hope and commitment as fundamental to understanding moral enterprises.

8. Minimizing Moral Losses

There will be times when we cannot alleviate the moral losses stemming from our choices. Suppose, for example, that we can wrong the dead and that routine retrieval, presumed consent, and familial consent will disrespect some dead persons. In that case, if we implement routine retrieval, presumed consent, or familial consent, we cannot alleviate the loss resulting from disrespecting the dead. Once we violate their prior wishes by either taking their organs without consent or by allowing family members to override their prior wish to donate, we cannot do anything to correct or soften the wrong. We cannot apologize to the dead; we cannot provide them with any compensatory award; and no ritual, whether secular or religious, could soften the violation. The point is moot if we cannot wrong the dead.

Even if we cannot wrong the dead, we still face conflicts if the public believes that we can wrong the dead. We might try to avoid some conflicts involving routine retrieval by working to shape public opinion to accept or tolerate the practice. We could show, as people have, how retrieving corneas has helped many blind people to see. Those defending routine retrieval could argue that dead persons have no interests. If enough people accepted routine retrieval, we would not have to worry about ignoring or violating the preferences of those who object to the policy. Conversely, in a community where many individuals choose not to donate, routine retrieval is likely to be successful if and only if the public remains unaware of the practice.

A few years ago, journalist Connie Chung investigated routine retrieval of corneas in the United States for the American television news program "20/20." Her interviews with family members revealed their frustration when they learned about the removal of their loved one's corneas. Although people's emotions cannot always dictate policy, consideration of people's emotions is a large part of taking a justifiable moral stance. In the case of the routine removal of corneas, we cannot alleviate or avoid the loss of disturbing those family members.

Presumed consent would also be controversial, but not as controversial as routine retrieval. Are there steps we could take to avoid or alleviate the losses of implementing presumed consent? We could make the opting-out process easy, thereby avoiding the apparent moral loss of wronging the dead by violating their prior wishes. An easy opting-out process would also avoid the potential backlash of the public disapproving of the policy. There would be those who do not want their organs taken but never explicitly indicate their wish not to donate. In these cases, whether we believe presumed consent produces moral losses would depend, in part, on how we judge taking organs from those who had an easy opportunity to opt out but failed to do so.

Many individuals across the globe find the higher brain definition of death implausible. We may wonder, then, what would happen if we adopted the higher brain definition regardless of their beliefs. If we plan to implement the higher brain definition of death, we have a moral obligation to conduct public discussions. Otherwise, the transplant and medical community would suffer a predictable backlash, thereby jeopardizing the present level of public support for transplantation.

People care about these issues and need to be educated so they can develop informed opinions. The scientific-medical-bioethical community in different countries could try to convince the lay public to adopt the higher brain definition of death, but they must convince themselves first. Is this likely? I doubt it. This issue, like many others, questions our psychological malleability. Our attitudes toward the moral status of the dead and the definition of death can shift, but we should not underestimate the depth of many persons' beliefs that the permanent loss of higher brain functions does not constitute death and that we should treat the dead with respect.

The cardiopulmonary definition of death would lead to the retrieval of few organs for the immediate future, unless we reject the Dead Donor Rule. Rejecting the Dead Donor Rule or adopting more policies like the Pittsburgh protocol would not lead to a slippery slope in which members of transplant teams would kill living persons who are not seriously compromised to obtain their organs. We can establish institutional checks and balances to protect patients. The transplant community is not malicious. But this move creates other problems.

Rejecting the Dead Donor Rule allows the killing of some patients for their organs. Even with seriously compromised patients, this proposal would result in two forms of moral loss. It would result in the loss of killing those persons, and it diminishes our respect for life.

Obviously, we cannot alleviate the loss of killing persons. We could make a psychological adjustment by convincing ourselves as Truog has that such killing is justified. Reverence for a high quality life apparently motivates Truog to abandon the Dead Donor Rule. The problem is that such a psychological adjustment is also symptomatic of a loss of respect for life and a cause for further eroding respect. Like routine retrieval, alleviating, or avoiding some moral losses from implementing a higher brain definition or abandoning the Dead Donor Rule are impossible.

As for selling organs, I believe most people would prefer financial remuneration for their organs that surgeons would retrieve after they die. But this is only a guess. In contrast, I think the American public would have a more difficult time believing that retrieving organs from living sellers is justified. Social scientists can help us with anticipating the public's attitudes, thereby allowing us to understand people's preferences and to anticipate their emotional responses to organ sales. We must consider, though, whether we could alleviate other problems with moral losses stemming from organ sales.

Selling organs would undermine the sense of community that the altruistic tradition fosters. Can we do anything to alleviate this problem? When considering live-organ sales, we must try to assess whether we can properly honor our bodies and the bodies of others in an environment where we allow people to sell their own flesh and blood. We could not restore or alleviate the moral losses of commodifying the human body, if we allowed live organ sales.

With xenotransplantation, we can alleviate or avoid some of the conflicts. We would need to alleviate the pain and suffering of xenotransplant patients and minimize disease transmission to third parties. The medical-scientific community could alleviate the pain and suffering of xenotransplant patients by being honest about the prospects of their research and experimental therapies. This would spare early xenotransplant recipients and their families from being too hopeful. In this way, patients could find meaning in contributing to science and to the health of future patients. Even though the patients would suffer, they would know that they are suffering for a reason, and they would know that transplant surgeons have provided realistic information about their prospects for survival.

Through bioengineering and screening for viruses, we could limit problems with organ rejection and with transmitting diseases to the subject-patient and to third parties. Although I do not support the xenotransplantation of whole organs, proceeding cautiously through clinical trials reduces the risk of disaster. These safety measures minimize the probability of transmitting harmful bacteria and viruses to human beings but not enough to justify the xenotransplantation of whole organs.

We can do nothing to alleviate the loss of the animals sacrificed. Although I believe most of the global community would embrace xenotransplants if they proved successful, we would lose the value of pigs' lives. That we slaughter pigs for food does not alleviate that fact. We could make their lives as comfortable and enjoyable as possible and make their deaths as painless as possible. Although we are accustomed to killing animals for several purposes, justifying such killing remains problematic.

Stem cell research is promising, but technical and moral problems remain. Although the moral status of early embryos is contentious, there is growing support for embryonic stem cell research. To alleviate moral disagreements and political antagonisms, we need to educate citizens about the issue of moral status and about the biology of a blastocyst. Such efforts can foster understanding, respect for opposing views, and more moral agreement.

9. Conclusion

Commentators on the ethics of organ retrieval do not analyze routine retrieval, presumed consent, the definition of death, selling organs, xenotransplantation, or stem cell research in a vacuum independent of other strategies. Yet ethicists have not adequately explored the broad range of plausible possibilities for responding to people with failing or failed organs. For example, Amir Halevy and Baruch Brody contend that the whole brain definition undermines retrieval and transplant goals. The Committee on Xenografts suggests that xenotransplantation is necessary to meet the goals of transplantation. David K. C. Cooper and Robert Lanza make the point for xenotransplantation explicit when they assert that, "the need for transplantation is clear."[3]

Choosing to implement or reject a policy will have significant moral consequences but only in the context of many other decisions. We have seen that many ways exist to adjust for the number of transplantable organs. The many ways that we can change the number of available transplantable organs makes our options interesting, difficult to compare, and open-ended.

Adjusting to conflicts requires us to compare conflicting values. We cannot always assert with confidence whether values are commensurable, or whether our efforts at implementing retrieval strategies will be successful. With many of our decisions, we cannot tally the most probable overall balance of benefits and burdens, because outcomes depend upon present and future efforts. We should not expect a method or sharpened moral intuitions to indicate what actions will most likely produce the best outcome. Instead, we need a commitment to strategies in which we make a series of justified decisions that include adjustments to alleviate the negative results of choices between conflicting values and to build upon the value of paths selected.

At times, there will be best solutions we need to discover. Other times, we will have to resign ourselves to choosing a plausible path and doing the best we can. At times, we need to change our moral perspective from one in which we look for the best choice to one where we are committed to doing well with a good choice.

My approach leaves us with a tension between trying to find the best possible solution and acknowledging the incommensurability of some options. That is the challenge of taking incommensurability seriously. Thinking in terms of series of actions allows us to consider a broad range of plausible courses of actions, the ramifications of those actions, and the adjustments and commitments we must make to protect and secure values.

CONCLUSION

> In rare and isolated instances, it may really be the case that such a will to truth, some extravagant and adventurous courage, a metaphysician's ambition to hold a hopeless position, may participate and ultimately prefer even a handful of "certainty" to a whole carload of beautiful possibilities.[1]

We cannot eliminate value conflicts from the moral life. Conflicts like Sophie's can be so horrible and intractable that philosophers raise the possibility of persons facing incompatible moral requirements, quintessential dilemmas. Although the existence of dilemmas remains contentious, we often face conflicts that leave us with moral losses and residual moral requirements and reasons to alleviate the harm resulting from our choices, even when we choose well or optimally. The previous chapters illustrated interesting but troublesome residue-producing conflicts related to organ retrieval. I will end with some general remarks about regarding much of the moral life as a constructive process and achievement.

Commentators in applied ethics naturally ask us to support or reject proposed actions and policies. At times, our best policy decisions rest, in part, on vague hopes and judgments. People may agree with Hugo Tristram Engelhardt that moral conflicts are irresolvable by appeal to reason. In the end, we must choose among our options. The usual method for deciding an issue in applied ethics calls for accumulating relevant facts, identifying the values involved, prioritizing any conflicting values, factoring in the probabilities that possible acts could be accomplished, and then rendering a judgment. Although this method includes necessary features of good decision-making, I do think such an approach to applied ethics has us overlook the process of *constructing* good as a central feature of the moral life.

In one sense, we cannot deny the role of the constructive process in living morally. Organ retrieval and transplantation requires creative scientists, physicians, policy makers, mental health professionals, nurses, administrators, and ethicists who work to retrieve more organs, to protect the autonomy of donors and recipients, and to ensure good medicine and rehabilitation. We can all agree that successful organ transplantation is the result of a long process of conflict-ridden constructive efforts.

Conflicts may involve commensurable or incommensurable values. Commensurable value conflicts afford us the opportunity to discover and realize the most heavily weighted value. I have argued against implementing strategies such as routine retrieval and the xenotransplantation of whole organs. These judgments imply that I trust the possibility of accurate comparisons among some conflicting values. Even when we act upon and realize the highest value, we must face moral requirements or reasons to alleviate the moral loss of the value that we sacrificed. Making the right choice in times of conflict requires intelligence and sensitivity. To avoid, limit, or end the damage of unrealized values requires creativity. We have ample evidence that professionals involved with organ retrieval and transplantation often make adjustments with the aim of realizing value and limiting losses.

The incommensurability of some of the conflicting values prevents us from discovering a single best course of action to take, or a single best set of strategies. The need to make continuous interventions to bring about valuable results also leaves the ultimate outcome of strategies open ended, thereby contributing to the incommensurability of strategies and sets of strategies. Still, even incommensurable value conflicts lend themselves to rational deliberation. Assessing incommensurable values in a broader context of a series of decisions enables us to embark on a reasonable and justifiable course. In this way, rational sense can be made of an otherwise arbitrary decision between incommensurable conflicting values. Rational deliberation in these contexts is possible because even where value conflicts are incommensurable different actions can be justified as part of a series of actions aiming to realize values while limiting the damage resulting from the decisions. This point is significant and warrants clarification.

Once we make a decision, we often appropriately make adjustments to avoid conflicts and losses resulting from that choice. The Pittsburgh protocol, for example, allows us to adopt a cardiopulmonary definition of death and to retrieve more organs without abandoning the Dead Donor Rule. We should recall that accepting Pittsburgh's protocol compels us to make another controversial conceptual adjustment—to accept death as reversible.

In their attempt to overcome a transplant recipient's immune response, scientists are genetically engineering pigs to make xenotransplantation safer. We can also make legal and institutional adjustments to accommodate the sale of organs. We cannot always predict the moral fallout of such adjustments; to conclude with certainty that the implementation of some policies is justified is not possible. The consequences of implementing a policy are morally relevant. Those consequences depend upon future successes and failures. In turn, future successes and failures depend upon the present decisions we make. For example, rejecting xenotransplantation will give us reason to pursue other avenues such as organ sales, stem cell research, and better preventive medicine. Doubtless, our level of commitment contributes to whether a venture will prove successful.

Abandoning the possibility of moral discoveries in the context of choosing among incommensurable alternatives provides explanatory room for understanding much of our moral behavior. If we are not making discoveries when making decisions regarding the morality of organ retrieval strategies, what are we doing? Are we foolishly trying to discover values that are not there? Are we merely expressing intersubjective whims? Perhaps we are riding out the cultural inertia produced by the diverging forces of religion and science. Alternatively, do we ride the coattails of dynamic personalities who convert others to their point of view? Different interpretations possess elements of truth. If I am right, much of what we do is constructively adjust our concepts, laws, attitudes, institutions, and technologies in the attempt to realize widely shared values and to alleviate the fallout from conflicts.

Instead of insisting upon there being discoverable moral answers to every moral question, we should embrace our constructive possibilities in moral matters. This approach enables us to evaluate our choices and stimulates us to question our boundaries and values while simultaneously reaffirming and strengthening our commitment to some values. It also gives us the conceptual wherewithal to be flexible without breaking. The question is how malleable are we as individuals, societies, and a global community? How malleable is the moral life? To answer these questions, we should gain a sense of the ways in which we construct our moral lives.

I do not mean to give the impression that we construct moral lives with a fixed set of values, as if constructing a moral life mirrors cooking in the sense that intrinsic values constitute the moral ingredients that can be combined in different ways to make a good life. We may wonder whether we construct the values themselves. I am not asking whether we construct values out of nothing. I assume that we do not. But why not think of all of our values as something we construct based upon our needs, purposes, and limitations instead of as discoveries of the moral life? Impressive philosophers such as John Leslie Mackie and Patricia Greenspan have argued that we create moral concepts to suit our individual and collective purposes.[2]

A thoughtful sincere person might think that my presentation of constructive pluralism and the views of Mackie and Greenspan share some similar flaws. Others may find the idea of constructing our values to be misleading and perhaps even disturbing. The fear of thinking that we create all of our values stems from reluctance to believe that we can do well without valuing autonomy, pleasure, respect for persons, loyalty, love, justice, and so forth. What many hold to be intrinsic values may be merely instrumental values to suit identified purposes. Is this fear justified?

Philosophers may disagree over the number and types of intrinsic values. While this does not mean that they will often disagree as to which actions, events, attitudes, objects, and subjects are valuable, in some cases they might. People passionately disagree over the intrinsic value of pigs, embryos, fetuses, the dead, and those who are alive but lack a qualitatively meaningful life.

Prima facie, some of these disagreements result from a disagreement regarding the types of intrinsic values under consideration, because values support our views over who has moral status. Some disagreements stem from differences as to how to rank conflicting values, and whether psychological, religious, or political values can override moral values. A commitment to a list of intrinsic values can make it difficult to explain why some entities are valuable.

We have seen, for example, the difficulty of arguing why the dead, the nearly dead, many animals, and embryos and fetuses should be valued if we accept familiar values such as respect for persons, pleasure, and self-realization. What we regard as our values does not allow us to fully understand many of our moral intuitions and responses. For this reason, we might construct a better system of values—one that will cohere better with common moral intuitions and responses. At times, this will mean we need to change our moral principles; other times, we will need to revise our intuitive judgments.

To address the gaps in our moral thinking we must consider several options. First, we can add to the list of intrinsic values so that we include entities such as the dead, the nearly dead, animals, embryos, and fetuses under our moral umbrella. A convincing list of values could help quell debates over the intrinsic value of such entities. Second, we can reconceptualize traditional lists of values until they render the logical consequences needed to explain more of our moral intuitions. For example, we must better understand what it means to value human life. Third, we can adjust our moral intuitions to fit with the consequences of familiar lists of values. If we take that option, we might regard the value that many of us place on the dead and the nearly dead with suspicion if not derision.

We can engage in many conceptual maneuverings. When we think that we can construct values in the sense of developing concepts that help us lead good lives, rethinking those values when they fail to guide our actions in many cases or when they suggest we perform actions that we find counterintuitive, then we should feel less threatened.

Moral boundaries limit us as to the way we can reconfigure our lists of values and the way we conceptualize those values. Every moral framework must count some actions as valuable all other things remaining equal: saving qualitatively meaningful lives, the prevention and amelioration of extreme suffering, and the protection of liberties. Conversely, every moral framework must count some actions as immoral all other things being equal. The routine murder of healthy individuals for their organs is but one example. Improving our moral belief system will not eliminate all conflicts; that is just the way of the world. We can reasonably respond to these conflicts even if we do not always agree as to what is the best solution to a problem. We address the conflicts by acknowledging the complexity, making a justified decision, and making adjustments to avoid more conflicts or to alleviate the moral losses. At times, that is the best we can do.

Ultimately, my analysis of our quest for organs makes the following points. First, the quest for organs is a broad moral project affected by many policy decisions, the weighing of values, many adjustments, and belief in the potential of developing medical technologies. Second, it shows that our moral options are much more open ended than suggested by dilemmas, whether the dilemmas are real or merely apparent. The overall moral balance of our choices will depend upon a host of efforts that extend through time.

Decisions must include identifying and comparing conflicting values, and be part of an overall program to make the world a better place—a program that requires hope, luck, commitment, and a willingness to change strategies. Trivial decisions will only involve a small cluster of actions that do not significantly affect our future; significant or momentous decisions will involve a large cluster of actions that may extend indefinitely, large enough so that no one will be able to anticipate all of the outcomes and possible options. We must resist thinking that we only need to imagine a variety of possibilities and then, based on the mix of facts, values, and probabilities, make the decision that maximizes value. The problem with this thinking is twofold. We cannot project far enough into the future about likely outcomes, and the probabilities of different outcomes are contingent upon present and future efforts, and luck.

The usual presumption in applied ethics is that we can find a single best response to moral problems, especially when discussing a conflict within a cultural context. Often, this may be so. But many moral problems do not have a unique best response. Even when a best response exists, our limitations may prevent our knowing it.

Not everyone believes that we should expect to find unique answers to complex moral issues facing applied ethicists. Scholars typically explain our failure to find unique answers with theories of cultural or moral relativism, cultural or moral pluralism, nihilism, or fuzzy moral intuitions. There may be merit in all of these explanations, but none explains all of the disagreements. Medical ethics scholars frequently underestimate the problem of incommensurability and virtually always fail to consider the constructive nature of morality as an alternative explanation for our inability to establish the best route to take in some cases. Viewing morality as a constructive process allows us to stop looking for a single solution to complex problems involving conflicting values and to choose among several plausible paths, all of which require or give reasons to make adjustments to protect and ensure the realization of values.

My account is radically pluralistic in that even people of the same culture in the same circumstances can respond to some moral problems with different, yet justified responses. My account does not tell us whether we ought to be conservative or pioneering with our moral projects. It does emphasize the wide range of our moral possibilities while also recognizing moral boundaries. We should continue efforts to help transplant candidates, but not at the risk of undermining values fundamental to a good society. We must pull in the reins on some strategies and technological developments, a commitment that may be the most challenging adjustment the global community needs to make.

NOTES

Introduction

1. OPTN: The Organ Procurement and Transplant Network is a source for these and many other data regarding donor organ availability, transplant waiting lists, and survival rates. URL = < http:www.OPTN.org> accessed 11 January 2005.

2. Terrance C. McConnell, "Moral Residue and Dilemmas," *Moral Dilemmas and Moral Theory*, ed. H. E. Mason (New York: Oxford University Press, 1996), pp. 36–47.

3. Tom L. Beauchamp and James F. Childress, *Principles of Biomedical Ethics*, 4th ed. (New York: Oxford University Press, 1994).

4. Edmund D. Pellegrino and David C. Thomasma, *The Virtues in Medical Practice* (New York: Oxford University Press, 1993).

5. Albert R. Jonsen, Mark Siegler, and William J. Winslade, *Clinical Ethics: A Practical Approach to Ethical Decisions in Clinical Medicine*, 4th ed. (New York: McGraw-Hill, 1998).

6. H. Tristram Engelhardt, *The Foundations of Bioethics*, 2nd ed. (New York: Oxford University Press, 1996).

7. Beauchamp and Childress, *Principles of Biomedical Ethics*, pp. 20–23.

8. Rosemarie Tong, *Feminist Approaches to Bioethics: Theoretical Reflections and Practical Applications* (Boulder, Colo.: Westview Press, 1997).

9. Engelhardt, *Foundations of Bioethics*, pp. 12, 35, 47, 127.

10. Elizabeth Anderson, *Value in Ethics and Economics* (Cambridge Mass.: Harvard University Press, 1993).

11. Raymond Gillespie Frey, "Conflict and Resolution: On Values and Trade-Offs," *Social Policy and Conflict Resolution*, eds. Thomas Attig, Donald Callen, and Raymond Gillespie Frey (Bowling Green, Ohio: Applied Philosophy Program, Bowling Green State University, 1984), pp. 1–16.

12. Robert Truog, "Is It Time to Abandon Brain Death?" *Hastings Center Report* (January–February 1997), pp. 29–37.

13. Robert M. Veatch, "The Impending Collapse of the Whole Brain Definition of Death," *Hastings Center Report* (July–August 1993), p. 23.

14. H. Tristram Engelhardt, "Reexamining the Definition of Death and Becoming Clearer about What It Is to Be Alive," *Death: Beyond Whole Brain Criteria*, ed. Richard M. Zaner (Dordrecht, Holland: Kluwer, 1988), pp. 91–98.

15. Committee on Xenograft Transplantation: Ethical Issues and Public Policy, *Xenotransplantation: Science, Ethics, and Public Policy*, ed. Division of Health Sciences Policy, Division of Healthcare Services, Institute of Medicine (Washington, D.C.: National Academy Press, 1996).

16. Ruth Barcan Marcus, "Moral Dilemmas and Consistency," *Journal of Philosophy*, 77 (1980), pp. 121–136.

17. See Thomas Nagel, "The Fragmentation of Value," *Mortal Questions* (New York: Cambridge University Press, 1979), pp. 73–74; and Susan Wolf, "Two Levels of Pluralism," *Ethics*, 102 (July 1992), pp. 720–742.

Chapter One

1. Aristotle, *Nicomachean Ethics* (Indianapolis, Ind.: Hackett Publishing Company, 1985), 3.13 30–110b.

2. William Styron, *Sophie's Choice* (New York: Bantam Books, 1980).

3. Peter Railton, "Pluralism, Determinacy, and Dilemma," *Ethics*, 102 (July 1992), pp. 720–742.

4. Terrance C. McConnell, "Moral Residue and Dilemmas," *Moral Dilemmas and Moral Theory*, ed. H. E. Mason (New York: Oxford University Press, 1996), pp. 36–47.

5. Patricia S. Greenspan, "Moral Dilemmas and Guilt," *Philosophical Studies*, 43 (1983), pp. 117–125.

6. Ibid., p. 119.

7. Jeremy Bentham, *An Introduction to the Principles of Morals and Legislation* (New York: Oxford University Press, 1823).

8. Immanuel Kant, *Grounding for the Metaphysics of Morals*, trans. James W. Ellington (Indianapolis, Ind.: Hackett Publishing Company, 1981).

9. William David Ross, *The Right and the Good* (New York: Oxford University Press, 1930).

10. Charles Taylor, "The Diversity of Goods," *Utilitarianism and Beyond*, eds. Amartya Sen and Bernard Williams (New York: Cambridge University Press, 1982), pp. 129–144.

11. Michael Stocker, *Plural and Conflicting Values* (Oxford, England: Clarendon Press, 1990).

12. Fred Feldman, "On the Intrinsic Value of Pleasures," *Ethics*, 107 (April 1997), pp. 448–466.

13. Isaiah Berlin, "Two Concepts of Liberty," *Four Essays on Liberty* (New York: Oxford University Press, 1969).

14. McConnell, "Moral Residue and Dilemmas," p. 36.

15. Bernard Williams, *Moral Luck* (New York: Cambridge University Press, 1981).

16. Ross, *The Right and the Good*, p. 28.

17. David O. Brink, "Moral Conflict and Its Structure," *Moral Dilemmas and Moral Theory*, ed. H. E. Mason (New York: Oxford University Press, 1996), pp. 102–104.

18. Williams, *Moral Luck*, p. 73.

19. Ibid., pp. 73–74.

20. Ibid., p. 73.

21. Brink, "Moral Conflict and Its Structure," p. 114.

22. Mary Mothersill, "The Moral Dilemmas Debate," *Moral Dilemmas and Moral Theory*, ed. H. E. Mason (New York: Oxford University Press, 1996), pp. 66–85.

23. Brink, "Moral Conflict and Its Structure," pp. 115–116.

24. Thomas Nagel, "The Fragmentation of Value," *Mortal Questions* (New York: Cambridge University Press, 1979), pp. 73–74

25. Bas C. van Fraassen, "Values and the Heart's Command," *Moral Dilemmas*, ed. Christopher Gowans (New York: Oxford University Press, 1987), p. 144.

26. Alan Donagan, "Consistency in Rationalist Moral Systems," *Moral Dilemmas*, ed. Christopher Gowans (New York: Oxford University Press, 1987), pp. 285–286.

27. Greenspan, "Moral Dilemmas and Guilt," p. 124n5.

28. Thomas Hill, "Moral Dilemmas, Gaps, and Residues: A Kantian Perspective," *Moral Dilemmas and Moral Theory*, ed. H. E. Mason (New York: Oxford Uni-

versity Press, 1996), pp. 167–199.

29. Ibid., p. 176.

30. Walter Sinnott-Armstrong, *Moral Dilemmas* (Oxford: Basil Blackwell, 1988), pp. 216–233.

31. Frithjof Bergmann, "A Monologue on the Emotions," *Understanding Human Emotions* (Bowling Green, Ohio: Bowling Green Studies in Applied Philosophy, 1979), esp. pp. 3–8.

32. Ibid., pp. 5–8.

33. McConnell, "Moral Residue and Dilemmas," p. 38.

34. Ibid.

35. Ibid.

36. Ibid., p. 39.

37. Ibid.

38. Walter Sinnott-Armstrong, "Moral Dilemmas and Rights," *Moral Dilemmas and Moral Theory*, ed. H. E. Mason (New York: Oxford University Press, 1996), p. 55.

39. Patricia S. Greenspan, *Practical Guilt: Moral Dilemmas, Emotions, and Social Norms* (New York: Oxford University Press, 1995).

40. Ibid., p. 152.

41. Ibid.

42. Sinnott-Armstrong, *Moral Dilemmas*, p. 50.

43. Ibid., pp. 11–22.

44. Ibid., pp. 216–220.

45. Donagan, "Consistency in Rationalist Moral Systems," p. 282.

46. Ibid., p. 285.

47. McConnell, "Moral Residue and Dilemmas," p. 41.

48. Ibid., p. 43.

49. Ibid., p. 41.

Chapter Two

1. *The Decision: Whose Kidney Is It Anyway?* FFH 6438 (Princeton, N.J.: Films for the Humanities & Sciences, 1996), film.

2. David Price, *Legal and Ethical Aspects of Organ Transplantation* (New York: Cambridge University Press, 2000), p. 249.

3. Tom L. Beauchamp and James F. Childress, *Principles of Biomedical Ethics*, 4th ed. (New York: Oxford University Press, 1994).

4. Ibid., pp. 29–30.

5. Ibid., p. 32.

6. Ibid., p. 31.

7. Ibid.

8. Ibid.

9. Ibid., p. 32.

10. Ibid., p. 3.

11. Ibid., p. 10

12. Ibid., p. 16.

13. Ibid., p. 17.

14. Ibid.

15. Ibid.

16. John Rawls, *A Theory of Justice* (Cambridge, Mass.: Harvard University Press, 1971), pp. 48–51.

17. Beauchamp and Childress, *Principles of Biomedical Ethics*, p. 21.

18. Ibid., p. 22.

19. Ibid.

20. Ibid., p. 28.

21. Ibid., p. 18.

22. Edmund D. Pellegrino and David C. Thomasma, *The Virtues in Medical Practice* (New York: Oxford University Press, 1993), p. 188.

23. Ibid., p. 19.

24. Albert R. Jonsen, Mark Siegler, and William J. Winslade, *Clinical Ethics: A Practical Approach to Ethical Decisions in Clinical Medicine*, 4th ed. (New York: McGraw-Hill, 1998).

25. Pellegrino and Thomasma, *The Virtues in Medical Practice*, pp. xi, 20–95.

26. Ibid., p. 20.

27. Ibid., p. 59.

28. Ibid.

29. Ibid., p. 55.

30. Ibid., p. 89.

31. Ibid.

32. Ibid., p. 87.

33. Carol Gilligan, *In a Different Voice: Psychological Theory and Women's Development* (Cambridge, Mass.: Harvard University Press, 1982).

34. Rosemarie Tong, *Feminist Approaches to Bioethics: Theoretical Reflections and Practical Applications* (Boulder, Colo.: Westview Press, 1997).

35. Ibid., p. 95.

36. Susan Sherwin, *No Longer Patient: Feminist Ethics & Healthcare* (Philadelphia, Pa.: Temple University Press, 1992), pp. 51–89.

37. Ibid., p. 92.

38. Ibid., p. 94.

39. Ibid., p. 82.

40. Ibid., p. 89.

41. Jonsen, Siegler, and Winslade, *Clinical Ethics*, p. 2.

42. Ibid.. p. 9.

43. Ibid.

44. Ibid., p. 157.

45. Ibid., p. 89.

46. Ibid., p. 48.

47. Ibid.

48. Ibid., pp. 77–78.

49. Ibid., p. 79.

50. Ibid.

51. H. Tristram Engelhardt, *The Foundations of Bioethics*, 2nd ed. (New York: Oxford University Press, 1996), p. 9

52. H. Tristram Engelhardt, *Bioethics and Secular Humanism: The Search for a Common Morality* (Laurel, Md.: Trinity Press International, 1991), p. 104.

53. Engelhardt, *Foundations of Bioethics*, p. 9.

54. Ibid., p. 74.

55. Engelhardt, *Bioethics and Secular Humanism*, p. xiv.
56. Ibid., p. 3.
57. Engelhardt, *Foundations of Bioethics*, p. 421.
58. Engelhardt, *Bioethics and Secular Humanism*, pp. 104–105.
59. Engelhardt, *Foundations of Bioethics*, p. 58.
60. Engelhardt, *Bioethics and Secular Humanism*, p. 15.
61. Engelhardt, *Foundations of Bioethics*, pp. 41–42.
62. Ibid., pp. 4–5, 35.
63. Ibid., p. 73.
64. Ibid., p. 75.

Chapter Three

1. Susan Wolf, "Two Levels of Pluralism," *Ethics*, 102 (July 1992), pp. 785–798.
2. Peter Railton, "Pluralism, Determinacy, and Dilemma," *Ethics*, 102 (July 1992), pp. 720–742.
3. John Stuart Mill, *Utilitarianism* (Indianapolis, Ind.: Hackett Publishing Company, 1979).
4. Brad Hooker, "Ross Style Pluralism versus Rule-Consequentialism," *Mind*, 105 (October 1996), p. 540.
5. Ibid.
6. Lawrence C. Becker, "Places for Pluralism," *Ethics*, 102 (July 1992), pp. 707–719.
7. Wolf, "Two Levels of Pluralism," p. 788.
8. Elizabeth Anderson, *Value in Ethics and Economics* (Cambridge Mass.: Harvard University Press, 1993); Wolf, "Two Levels of Pluralism"; and Michael Stocker, *Plural and Conflicting Values* (Oxford, England: Clarendon Press, 1990).
9. Wolf, "Two Levels of Pluralism," pp. 788–789.
10. John Kekes, *The Morality of Pluralism* (Princeton, N.J.: Princeton University Press, 1993).
11. Ibid., chap. 3.
12. Ibid., p. 26.
13. Wolf, "Two Levels of Pluralism," pp. 788–789.
14. Ibid., pp. 792–793.
15. Stocker, *Plural and Conflicting Values*, pp. 178–179.
16. William David Ross, *The Right and the Good* (New York: Oxford University Press, 1930), p. 30.
17. Thomas Nagel, *Mortal Questions* (New York: Cambridge University Press, 1979), p. 135.
18. Immanuel Kant, *Grounding for the Metaphysics of Morals*, trans. James W. Ellington (Indianapolis, Ind.: Hackett Publishing Company, 1981).
19. Aristotle, *Nicomachean Ethics* (Indianapolis, Ind.: Hackett Publishing Company, 1985), 3.13 30–110b.
20. Gerald H. Paske, "Genuine Moral Dilemmas and the Containment of Incoherence," *The Journal of Value Inquiry*, 24:4 (October 1990), pp. 315–323.
21. Ruth Chang, "Introduction," *Incommensurability, Incomparability, and Practical Reason* (Cambridge, Mass.: Harvard University Press, 1997).

22. Matthew Lawrence, "Pluralism, Liberalism, and the Role of Overriding Values," *Pacific Philosophical Quarterly*, 77 (1996), pp. 335–350.

23. Chang, "Introduction," p. 2.

24. Anderson, *Value in Ethics and Economics*.

25. Ibid., p. 55.

26. Chang, "Introduction," pp. 4–5.

27. Elizabeth Anderson, "Practical Reason and Incommensurable Goods," *Incommensurability, Incomparability, and Practical Reason*, ed. Ruth Chang (Cambridge, Mass.: Harvard University Press, 1997), p. 99.

28. Terrance McConnell, "Dilemmas and Incommensurateness," *The Journal of Value Inquiry*, 27 (1993), pp. 247–252.

29. Ibid., p. 249.

30. James Griffin, "Are There Incommensurable Values?" *Philosophy & Public Affairs*, 7:1 (1977), pp. 39–59.

31. Raymond Gillespie Frey, "Conflict and Resolution: On Values and Trade-Offs," *Social Policy and Conflict Resolution*, eds. Thomas Attig, Donald Callen, and Raymond Gillespie Frey (Bowling Green, Ohio: Applied Philosophy Program, Bowling Green State University, 1984), pp. 1–16.

32. Ibid., p. 1.

33. Chang, "Introduction," p. 5.

34. Ibid., p. 6.

35. Ibid., p. 7.

36. Ibid., p. 14.

37. Ibid., pp. 14–17.

38. Anderson, "Practical Reason and Incommensurable Goods," pp. 102–103.

39. Chang, "Introduction," pp. 18–19.

40. James Griffin, "Incommensurability: What's the Problem?" *Incommensurability, Incomparability, and Practical Reason*, ed. Ruth Chang (Cambridge, Mass.: Harvard University Press, 1997), p. 37.

41. Chang, "Introduction," p. 21.

42. Ibid., pp. 21–22.

43. Donald Regan, "Value, Comparability, and Choice," *Incommensurability, Incomparability, and Practical Reason*, ed. Ruth Chang, (Cambridge, Mass.: Harvard University Press, 1997), pp. 129–150.

44. Griffin, "Incommensurability," pp. 40–41.

45. Anderson, "Practical Reason and Incommensurable Goods," p. 103.

46. Stocker, *Plural and Conflicting Values*, p. 201.

Chapter Four

1. Robert Berkow, ed., *The Merck Manual of Medical Information*, Home Edition (Whitehouse Station, N.J.: Merck Research Laboratories, 1997).

2. D. Joralemon, and K. M. Fujinaga, "Studying the Quality of Life after Organ Transplantation: Research Problems and Solutions," *Social Science & Medicine*, 44:9 (May 1997), pp. 1259–1269.

3. C. Littlefield, S. Abbey, D. Fiducia, et al., "Quality of Life Following Transplantation of the Heart, Liver, and Lungs," *General Hospital Psychiatry*, 18, Suppl. 6 (November 1996), pp. 36s–47s.

4. Ibid., p. 37s.

5. P. Salmon, G. Mikhail, S. C. Stanford, S. Zielinsk, and J. R. Pepper, "Psychological Adjustment after Cardiac Transplantation," *Journal of Psychosomatic Research*, 45:5 (November 1998), pp. 449–458.

6. Joralemon, "Studying the Quality of Life After Organ Transplantation," pp. 1261–1262.

7. J. C. Spann, and C. Van Meter, "Cardiac Transplantation," *Surgical Clinics of North America*, 78:5 (October 1998), pp. 679–690.

8. Ibid., p. 688.

9. R. Hetzer et al., "Status of Patients Presently Living 9 to 13 Years after Orthotopic Heart Transplantation," *Annals of Thoracic Surgery*, 64:6 (December 1997), pp. 1661–1668.

10. A. Jalowiec, K. L. Grady, C. White-Williams, S. Fazekas, M. Laff, V. Davidson-Bell, et al., "Symptom Distress Three Months after Heart Transplantation," *Journal of Heart & Lung Transplantation*, 16:6 (June 1997), p. 611.

11. K. L. Grady, A. Jalowiec, C. White-Williams, et al., "Quality of Life 6 Months After Heart Transplantation Compared With Indicators of Illness Severity Before Transplantation," *American Journal of Critical Care*, 7:2 (March 1998), pp. 114–115.

12. Spann and Van Meter, "Cardiac Transplantation," p. 688.

13. Jalowiec et al., "Symptom Distress Three Months after Heart Transplantation," p. 610.

14. Salmon et al., "Psychological Adjustment after Cardiac Transplantation," p. 455.

15. The Neoral Transplant Learning Center, *Your Heart Transplant—Every Step of the Way* (East Hanover, N.J.: Norvartis Pharmaceutical Corporation, 1997).

16. Z. M. Younossi and G. Guyatt, "Quality-of-Life Assessments and Chronic Liver Disease," *American Journal of Gastroenterology*, 93:7 (July 1998), pp. 1037–1041.

17. Elizabeth Jonsen, E. Athlin, and O. Suhr, "Familial Amyloidotic Patients' Experience of the Disease and of Liver Transplantation," *Journal of Advanced Nursing*, 27:1 (January 1998), pp. 52–58.

18. Younossi, "Quality-of-Life Assessments and Chronic Liver Disease," p. 1037.

19. R. E. Tarter, "Quality of Life Following Liver Transplantation," *Hepato-Gastroenterology*, 45:23 (September–October 1998), pp. 1398–1403.

20. C. R. Gross, M. Malinchoc, W. R. Kim, et al., "Quality of Life Before and After Liver Transplantation for Cholestatic Liver Disease," *Hepatology*, 29:2 (February 1999), pp. 356–364.

21. Jonsen, "Familial Amyloidotic Patients' Experience of the Disease and of Liver Transplantation," p. 53.

22. S. K. Geevarghese, A. E. Bradley, J. K. Wright, et al., "Outcomes Analysis in 100 Liver Transplantation Patients," *American Journal of Surgery*, 175:5 (May 1998), pp. 349–350.

23. Gross et al., "Quality of Life Before and After Liver Transplantation for Cholestatic Liver Disease," p. 362.

24. Jonsen, "Familial Amyloidotic Patients' Experience of the Disease and of Liver Transplantation," p. 56.

25. Gross et al., "Quality of Life Before and After Liver Transplantation for Cholestatic Liver Disease," p. 358.

26. United Network for Organ Sharing, URL = < http:www.OPTN.org> accessed 17 February 2005.

27. Mickie Hall Faris, *When Your Kidneys Fail* (Los Angeles, Calif.: National Kidney Foundation of Southern California, 1994), p. 8.

28. Arthur J. Matas, L. McHugh, W. D. Payne, L. E. Wrenshall, D. L. Dunn, R. W. Gruessner, D. E. Sutherland, and J. S. Najarian, "Long-Term Quality of Life after Kidney and Simultaneous Pancreas-Kidney Transplantation," *Clinical Transplantation*, 12:3 (June 1998), pp. 233–242.

29. G. Mingardi, "Quality of Life and End Stage Renal Disease," *International Journal of Artificial Organs*, 21:11 (November 1998), pp. 741–747.

30. R. Jofre, J. M. Lopez-Gomez, F. Moreno, D. Sanz-Guajardo, and F. Valderrabano, "Changes in Quality of Life after Renal Transplantation," *American Journal of Kidney Diseases*, 32:1 (July 1998), pp. 93–100; and F. Pisani, G. Vennarecci, G. Tisone, O. Buonomo, G. Iaria, S. Rossi, A. Famulari, and C. U. Casciani, "Quality of Life and Long-Term Follow-Up after Kidney Transplantation: A 30-Year Clinical Study," *Transplantation Proceedings*, 29:7 (November 1997), pp. 2812–2813.

31. Transplant Service of the University of Texas Medical Branch at Galveston, *Kidney Transplantation* (Galveston, Tex.: University of Texas, 1998), p. 4.

32. C. D. Johnson, "Racial and Gender Differences in Quality of Life Following Kidney Transplantation," *Image—The Journal of Nursing Scholarship*, 30:2 (1998), pp. 125–130.

33. Transplant Service of the University of Texas Medical Branch at Galveston, *Kidney Transplantation*.

Chapter Five

1. George Pitcher, "The Misfortunes of the Dead," *American Philosophical Quarterly*, 21:2 (April 1984), pp. 183–188; and Joel Feinberg, *Harm to Others: The Moral Limits of the Criminal Law* (New York: Oxford University Press, 1987).

2. Anthony Serafini, "Callahan 'On Harming the Dead'," *Journal of Philosophical Research*, 15 (1989–1990), p. 336.

3. Mary Anne Warren, *Moral Status: Obligations to Persons and Other Living Things* (New York: Oxford University Press, 2000).

4. Peter Singer, *Animal Liberation* (New York: Harper Collins, 1975).

5. Holmes Rolston III, "The Human Standing in Nature: Fitness in the Moral Overseer," *Values and Moral Standing*, eds. L. Wayne Sumner, Donald M Callen, and Thomas Attig (Bowling Green, Ohio: Applied Philosophy Program, Bowling Green State University, 1986), p. 8.

6. Robert M. Veatch, "Routine Inquiry about Organ Donation—An Alternative to Presumed Consent," *The New England Journal of Medicine*, 325:17 (24 October 1991), pp. 1246–1249.

7. Arthur L. Caplan, and Beth Virnig, "Is Altruism Enough?—Required Request and the Donation of Cadaveric Organs and Tissues in the United States," *Critical Care Clinics*, 6:4 (October 1990), pp. 1007–1018.

8. Council on Ethical and Judicial Affairs, American Medical Association, "Strategies for Cadaveric Organ Procurement: Mandated Choice and Presumed Consent," *Journal of the American Medical Association*, 272:10 (September 1994), pp. 809–812.

9. James F. Childress, "Ethical Criteria for Procuring and Distributing Organs for Transplantation," *Organ Transplantation Policy: Issues and Prospects*, eds. James F. Blumstein and Frank A Sloan (Durham, N.C.: Duke University Press, 1989), p. 98.

10. Feinberg, *Harm to Others*, pp. 45–46.

11. Ibid., p. 84.

12. Ibid.

13. Ibid., pp. 84–85.

14. Ibid., p. 87.

15. Pitcher, "The Misfortunes of the Dead," p. 186.

16. Ibid., p. 87.

17. Ibid., pp. 185–186; and Feinberg, *Harm to Others*, p. 90.

18. Feinberg, *Harm to Others*, p. 91.

19. Pitcher, "The Misfortunes of the Dead," pp. 183–184.

20. Ibid.

21. Ibid., p. 187; and Feinberg, *Harm to Others*, p. 91.

22. Pitcher, "The Misfortunes of the Dead," p. 188.

23. Feinberg, *Harm to Others*, p. 91.

24. Joan C. Callahan, "On Harming the Dead," *Ethics*, 97 (January 1987), p. 346.

25. Ibid., pp. 347–350.

26. Ibid., pp. 351–352.

27. Sarafini, "Callahan 'On Harming the Dead'," pp. 331, 338.

28. Ibid., p. 332.

29. Ibid., p. 337.

30. Ibid., p. 338.

31. William May, "Attitudes toward the Newly Dead," *The Hastings Center Studies*, 1:1 (1973), pp. 3–13.

32. Ibid.

33. Joel Feinberg, "The Mistreatment of Dead Bodies," *The Hastings Center Report*, 15:1 (February 1985), pp. 31–37.

34. Ibid., p. 35.

35. Ibid., p. 36.

36. Thomas L. O'Carroll, "Over My Dead Body: Recognizing Property Rights in Corpses," *Journal of Health and Hospital Law*, 29:4 (1997), pp. 238–256.

37. James F. Childress, "Organ and Tissue Procurement: Ethical and Legal Issues Regarding Cadavers," *Encyclopedia of Bioethics*, ed. Warren T. Reich (New York: Macmillan, 1996), pp. 1857–1865.

Chapter Six

1. Hans Jonas, *Philosophical Essays: From Ancient Creed to Technological Man* (Chicago, Ill.: The University of Chicago Press, 1974); and Amir Halevy and Baruch Brody, "Brain Death: Reconciling Definitions, Criteria, and Tests," *Annals of Internal Medicine*, 119:6, suppl.1 (15 September 1993), pp. 519–525.

2. Peter Singer, *Rethinking Life and Death: The Collapse of Our Traditional Ethics* (New York: St. Martin's Griffin, 1994), pp. 22–23.

3. Ibid., p. 24.

4. Ad Hoc Committee of the Harvard Medical School, "A Definition of Irreversible Coma," *Journal of the American Medical Association*, 205:6 (5 August 1968), pp. 337–340.

5. Ibid., p. 339.

6. President's Commission for the Study of Ethical Problems in Medicine and Biomedical and Behavioral Research, *Defining Death: A Report on the Medical, Legal and Ethical Issues in the Determination of Death* (Washington, D.C.: US GPO, July 1981), p. 5.

7. Ibid., p. 15.

8. Ibid., p. 33.

9. Ibid., pp. 34–38.

10. Ibid., p. 73.

11. Ibid., p. 2.

12. Ibid.

13. Laura A. Siminoff, and Alexia Bloch, "American Attitudes and Beliefs about Brain Death," *The Definition of Death: Contemporary Controversies*, eds. Stuart J. Youngner, Robert M. Arnold, and Renie Schapiro (Baltimore, Md.: The Johns Hopkins University Press, 1999), pp. 186–187.

14. Robert D. Truog and James C. Fackler, "Rethinking Brain Death," *Critical Care Medicine*, 20:12 (1992), pp. 1705–1713.

15. Robert M. Veatch, "The Impending Collapse of the Whole Brain Definition of Death," *Hastings Center Report* (July–August 1993), pp. 18–24.

16. Truog and Fackler, "Rethinking Brain Death," p. 1707.

17. Richard M. Zaner, "Brains and Persons: A Critique of Veatch's View," *Death: Beyond Whole Brain Criteria*, ed. Richard M. Zaner (Dordrecht, Holland: Kluwer, 1988), p. 7.

18. H. Tristram Engelhardt, "Reexamining the Definition of Death and Becoming Clearer about What It Is to Be Alive," *Death: Beyond Whole Brain Criteria*, ed. Richard M. Zaner (Dordrecht, Holland: Kluwer, 1988), p. 94

19. Robert Veatch, "Whole Brain, Neocortical, and Higher Brain Related Concepts," *Death Beyond Whole Brain Criteria*, ed. Richard M. Zaner (Dordrecht, Holland: Kluwer, 1988), p. 172.

20. Ibid., p. 16.

21. Ibid., p. 17.

22. Ibid.

23. Ibid.

24. Ibid., p. 18.

25. Ibid., p. 17.

26. Stuart J. Younger, statement made at a conference 25 June 1999 in Galveston, Tex.

27. Singer, *Rethinking Life and Death*, p. 31.

28. Veatch, "The Impending Collapse of the Whole Brain Definition of Death," pp. 21–22.

29. James L. Bernat, "A Defense of the Whole Brain Concept of Death," *Hastings Center Report*, 28:2 (March–April 1998), p. 22.

30. Robert M. Veatch, "The Definition of Death: Problems for Public Policy," *Dying: Facing the Facts*, 3rd ed., eds. Hannelore Wass, Robert A. Neimeyer, Felix, M Berardo, and Francis Taylor (New York: Taylor & Francis, 1995), p. 423; and *Death, Dying, and the Biological Revolution* (New Haven, Conn.: Yale University Press, 1989), p. 55.

31. Veatch, *Death, Dying, and the Biological Revolution*, p. 408.

32. Ibid.

33. Ibid., p. 55.

34. Ibid., p. 423.

35. Halevy and Brody, "Brain Death: Reconciling Definitions, Criteria, and Tests," p. 523.

36. Robert Truog, "Is It Time to Abandon Brain Death?" *Hastings Center Report* (January–February 1997), pp. 29–37.

37. Ibid.

38. Michael A. DeVita, and James V. Snyder, "Development of the University of Pittsburgh Medical Center Policy for the Care of Terminally Ill Patients Who May Become Organ Donors after Death Following the Removal of Life Support," *Kennedy Institute of Ethics Journal*, 3:2 (June 1993), p. 132.

39. Michael A. DeVita, James V. Snyder, and Ake Grenvik, "History of Organ Donation by Patients with Cardiac Death," *Kennedy Institute of Ethics Journal*, 3:2 (June 1993), p. 124.

40. Joanne Lynn, "Are the Patients Who Become Organ Donors under the Pittsburgh Protocol for 'Non-Heart-Beating Donors' Really Dead?" *Kennedy Institute of Ethics Journal*, 3:2 (June 1993), p. 169; and David Cole, "Statutory Definitions of Death and the Management of Terminally Ill Patients Who May Become Organ Donors After Death," *Kennedy Institute of Ethics Journal*, 3:2 (June 1993), p. 148.

41. David Lamb, "Reversibility and Death: A Reply to David J. Cole," *Journal of Medical Ethics*, 18:1 (1992), pp. 31–33.

42. Cole, "Statutory Definitions of Death," pp. 148–151.

43. Tom Tomlinson, "The Irreversibility of Death: Reply to Cole," *Kennedy Institute of Ethics Journal*, 3:2 (June 1993), pp. 161–162.

44. Renee C. Fox, "An Ignoble Form of Cannibalism: Reflections on the Pittsburgh Protocol for Procuring Organs from Non-Heart-Beating Cadavers," *Kennedy Institute of Ethics Journal*, 3:2 (June 1993), pp. 232–237.

45. Bernat, "A Defense of the Whole Brain Concept of Death," pp. 14–23.

46. Alan D. Shewmon, "Caution in the Definition and Diagnosis of Infant Brain Death," *Medical Ethics: A Guide for Health Professionals*, eds. John F. Monagle and David C. Thomasma (Gaithersburg, Md.: Aspen Publishers, 1988), pp. 38–57.

47. Bernat, "A Defense of the Whole Brain Concept of Death," p. 19.

48. Ibid.

49. Ibid., p. 22.

Chapter Seven

1. National Organ Transplant Act, Pub L No.98-507, 3 USC, 301, 1984.

2. Texas Anatomical Gift Act, Texas Health and Safety Code Ann. 692.001–92.016.

3. "Pennsylvania to Offer Incentive for Organ Donation," *Houston Chronicle*, 6 May 1999.

4. Ibid.

5. Ibid.

6. David J. Rothman, "The International Organ Traffic," *New York Review of Books* (26 March 1998), p. 15.

7. John Walter Edinger, "The Ethics of Organ Procurement" (PhD diss., The University of Texas at Austin, 1987).

8. Ibid., p. 67.

9. Laura A. Siminoff, R. M. Arnold, A. L. Caplan, B. A. Virnig, and D. L. Seltzer, "Public Policy Governing Organ and Tissue Procurement in the United States: Results from the National Organ and Tissue Procurement Study," *Annals of Internal Medicine*, 123:1 (1 July 1995), p. 10.

10. Edinger, *The Ethics of Organ Procurement*, p. 67.

11. Ibid., p. 68.

12. Amitai Etzioni, "Introduction: A Matter of Balance, Rights and Responsibilities," *The Essential Communitarian Reader* (Lanham, Md.: Rowman & Littlefield Publishers, Inc., 1998), pp. ix–xxiv.

13. Margaret Jane Radin, *Contested Commodities* (Cambridge, Mass.: Harvard University Press, 1996), p. xi.

14. Ibid., p. 42.

15. Ibid., p. xii.

16. Ibid., pp. 80–83.

17. Ibid., p. xiii.

18. Ibid., pp. 5–9.

19. Ibid., p. 79.

20. Ibid., pp. 103–105.

21. Ibid., p. 105.

22. Ibid., p. 125.

23. Ibid., pp. 125–126.

24. Ibid., p. 125.

25. Ibid., p. 126.

26. Rothman, "The International Organ Traffic," p. 15.

27. Ibid.

28. Gloria J. Banks, "Legal & Ethical Safeguards: Protection of Society's Most Vulnerable Participants in a Commercialized Organ Transplantation System," *American Journal of Law & Medicine*, 21:1 (1995), p. 81.

29. Renee C. Fox and Judith P. Swazey, "Leaving the Field," *Hastings Center Report* (September–October 1992).

30. Banks, "Legal & Ethical Safeguards," pp. 75–83.

31. Lloyd R. Cohen, "Increasing the Supply of Transplant Organs: The Virtues of a Futures Market," *George Washington Law Review*, 1:3 (1989).

32. Banks, "Legal & Ethical Safeguards," pp. 76–77.

33. Edmund Pellegrino, "Families' Self-Interest and the Cadaver's Organs: What Price Consent?" *The Ethics of Organ Transplants*, eds. Arthur L. Caplan and Daniel H. Coelho (Amherst, N.Y.: Prometheus Books, 1998), p. 206.

Chapter Eight

1. Committee on Xenograft Transplantation: Ethical Issues and Public Policy, *Xenotransplantation: Science, Ethics, and Public Policy*, ed. Division of Health Sciences Policy, Division of Healthcare Services, Institute of Medicine (Washington, D.C.: National Academy Press, 1996), p. 17.

2. Rebecca Malouin, "Surgeons' Quest for Life: The History and the Future of Xenotransplantation," *Perspectives in Biology and Medicine*, 37:3 (Spring 1994), pp. 416–428, esp. p. 418.

3. David K. C. Cooper, and Robert P. Lanza, *Xeno: The Promise of Transplanting Animal Organs Into Humans* (New York: Oxford University Press, 2000), p. 28.

4. Malouin, "Surgeons' Quest for Life," p. 418.

5. Cooper and Lanza, *Xeno*, p. 28.

6. Ibid., pp. 24–26.

7. Malouin, "Surgeons' Quest for Life," p. 418.

8. Cooper and Lanza, *Xeno*, p. 31.

9. Malouin, "Surgeons' Quest for Life," p. 419.

10. Ibid., esp. pp. 419–420.

11. Ibid., p. 421.

12. Peter Singer, *Rethinking Life and Death: The Collapse of Our Traditional Ethics* (New York: St. Martin's Griffin, 1994), pp. 164.

13. Cooper and Lanza, *Xeno,* p. 39.

14. Singer, *Rethinking Life and Death*, pp. 164–165.

15. Committee on Xenograft Transplantation, *Xenotransplantation*, pp. 13–14.

16. Harold Vanderpool, "Xenotransplantation: Progress and Promise," *Western Journal of Medicine*, 171 (November/December 1999), p. 333.

17. Committee on Xenograft Transplantation, *Xenotransplantation*, p. 49.

18. Ibid.

19. Cooper and Lanza, *Xeno*, pp. 53–54, 64.

20. Committee on Xenograft Transplantation*, Xenotransplantation*, p. 78.

21. Ray Gillespie Frey, "Medicine, Animal Experimentation, and the Moral Problem of Unfortunate Humans," *Social Philosophy & Policy Foundation* (New York: Cambridge University Press, 1996), pp. 181–211.

22. Ibid., p. 207.

23. Ibid., p. 199.

24. Jonathan Hughes, "Xenografting: Ethical Issues," *Journal of Medical Ethics*, 24 (1998), pp. 18–24.

25. Frey, "Medicine, Animal Experimentation, and the Moral Problem of Unfortunate Humans," p. 210.

26. A. S. Daar, "Ethics of Xenotransplantation: Animal Issues, Consent, and Likely Transformation of Transplant Ethics," *World Journal of Surgery*, 21 (1997), p. 976.

27. Committee on Xenograft Transplantation, *Xenotransplantation*, p. 42.

28. Ibid., p. 44.

29. Daar, "Ethics of Xenotransplantation," p. 977.

30. Ibid., p. 979.

31. Harold Vanderpool, "Commentary: A Critique of Clark's Frightening Xenotransplantation Scenario," *Journal of Law, Medicine & Ethics*, 27 (1999), p. 154.

32. Committee on Xenograft Transplantation, *Xenotransplantation*, p. 46.

33. Ibid.

34. Ibid., pp. 71–72.

35. Daar, "Ethics of Xenotransplantation," p. 977.

36. Ibid., pp. 977–979.

37. Ibid.

Chapter Nine

1. Maureen L. Condic, "The Basics about Stem Cells," *First Things*, no. 119 (January 2003), pp. 30–31.
2. Thomas B. Okarma, "Human Primordial Stem Cells," *Hastings Center Report*, 29:2 (March–April 1999), p. 30.
3. Ariane Sains, "The Stem Cell Frontier," *Europe* (April 2002), p. 28.
4. Geron Ethics Advisory Board, "Research with Human Embryonic Stem Cells: Ethical Considerations," *Hastings Center Report*, 29:2 (March–April 1999), p. 32.
5. John Fletcher, "Human Stem Cell Research: Continued Debate," *American Society for Bioethics and Humanities Exchange*, 2:2 (Spring 1999), p. 7.
6. Justin Gillis, "Adult Cells with Powers of Stem Cells are Reported," *Austin American Statesman*, 21 June 2002, p. A1.
7. Fletcher, "Human Stem Cell Research," pp. 2–7.
8. Ibid.
9. "Stem Cell Research Gets Backing," *Houston Chronicle*, 20 March 1999.
10. Geron Ethics Advisory Board, "Research with Human Embryonic Stem Cells."
11. Ibid., p. 32.
12. Glenn McGee and Arthur L. Caplan, "What's In the Dish?" *Hastings Center Report*, 29:2, p. 37.
13. Geron Ethics Advisory Board, "Research with Human Embryonic Stem Cells," p. 31.
14. Ibid., p. 33.
15. Lori P. Knowles, "Property, Progeny, and Patents," *Hastings Center Report* (March–April, 1999), p. 40.
16. Geron Ethics Advisory Board, "Research with Human Embryonic Stem Cells," p. 33.
17. Knowles, "Property, Progeny, and Patents," pp. 39–40.
18. Ibid.
19. Gladys B. White, "Foresight, Insight, Oversight," *Hastings Center Report*, 29:2 (March–April 1999), p. 42.
20. Fletcher, "Human Stem Cell Research," p. 7.
21. White, "Foresight, Insight, Oversight," p. 42.
22. Gillis, "Adult Cells with Powers of Stem Cells are Reported," pp. 1, 8.
23. Condic, "The Basics about Stem Cells," pp. 31–32.
24. Ibid., p. 33.
25. Ibid., p. 34.

Chapter Ten

1. Michael Stocker, *Plural and Conflicting Values* (Oxford, England: Clarendon Press, 1990).
2. Ruth Barcan Marcus, "Moral Dilemmas and Consistency," *Journal of Philosophy*, 77 (1980), pp. 121–136.
3. Terrance C. McConnell, "Moral Residue and Dilemmas," *Moral Dilemmas and Moral Theory*, ed. H. E. Mason (New York: Oxford University Press, 1996), pp. 44–45.
4. Mary Mothersill, "The Moral Dilemmas Debate," *Moral Dilemmas and Moral Theory*, ed. H. E. Mason (New York: Oxford University Press, 1996), p. 83.

5. Ibid.
6. Ibid., p. 82.
7. Renee C. Fox and Judith P. Swazey, *Spare Parts: Organ Replacement in American Society* (New York: Oxford University Press, 1992), p. 33.
8. Patricia S. Greenspan, *Practical Guilt: Moral Dilemmas, Emotions, and Social Norms* (New York: Oxford University Press, 1995), p. 142.
9. Michael Stocker, "Abstract and Concrete Value: Plurality, Conflict, and Maximization," in Ruth Chang, ed., *Incommensurability, Incomparability, and Practical Reasoning* (Cambridge, Mass.: Harvard University Press, 1997), p. 205; and Elizabeth Anderson, "Practical Reason and Incommensurable Goods," ibid., p. 94.

Chapter Eleven

1. Gerald H. Paske, "Genuine Moral Dilemmas and the Containment of Incoherence," *The Journal of Value Inquiry*, 24:4 (October 1990), pp. 315–323.
2. Terrance C. McConnell, "Moral Residue and Dilemmas," *Moral Dilemmas and Moral Theory*, ed. H. E. Mason (New York: Oxford University Press, 1996), p. 43.
3. David K. C. Cooper, and Robert P. Lanza, *Xeno: The Promise of Transplanting Animal Organs Into Humans* (New York: Oxford University Press, 2000).

Conclusion

1. Friedrich Nietzsche, *Beyond Good and Evil* (New York: Vintage Books, 1966).
2. J. L. Mackie, *Ethics: Inventing Right and Wrong* (New York: Penguin Books, 1977); and Patricia Greenspan, *Practical Guilt: Moral Dilemmas, Emotions, and Social Norms* (New York: Oxford University Press, 1995).

BIBLIOGRAPHY

Ad Hoc Committee of the Harvard Medical School. "A Definition of Irreversible Coma," *Journal of the American Medical Association,* 205 (August 1968), pp. 337–340.

Anderson, Elizabeth. "Practical Reason and Incommensurable Goods." In Chang. *Incommensurability, Incomparability, and Practical Reasoning.*

————. *Value in Ethics and Economics.* Cambridge, Mass.: Harvard University Press, 1993.

Aristotle. *Nichomachean Ethics.* Translated by Terence Irwin. Indianapolis, Ind.: Hackett Publishing Company, 1985.

Attig, Thomas, Donald Callen, and Raymond Gillespie Frey, eds. *Social Policy and Conflict Resolution.* Bowling Green, Ohio: Applied Philosophy Program, Bowling Green State University, 1984.

Banks, Gloria J. "Legal & Ethical Safeguards: Protection of Society's Most Vulnerable Participants in a Commercialized Organ Transplantation System," *American Journal of Law & Medicine,* 21:1 (1995), pp. 45–110.

Beauchamp, Tom L., and James F. Childress. *Principles of Biomedical Ethics,* 4th ed. New York: Oxford University Press, 1994.

Becker, Lawrence C. "Places for Pluralism," *Ethics,* 102 (July 1992), pp. 707–719.

Bentham, Jeremy. *An Introduction to the Principles of Morals and Legislation.* London: J. M. Creery, 1823.

Bergman, Frithjof. "A Monologue on the Emotions." In *Understanding Human Emotions.* Bowling Green, Ohio: Bowling Green Studies in Applied Philosophy, 1979.

Berkow, Robert, ed. The *Merck Manual of Medical Information.* Home ed. Whitehouse Station, N.J.: Merck Research Laboratories, 1997.

Berlin, Isaiah. "Two Concepts of Liberty." In *Four Essays on Liberty.* New York: Oxford University Press, 1969.

Bernat, James L. "A Defense of the Whole Brain Concept of Death," *Hastings Center Report,* 28:2 (1998), p. 22.

Blumstein, James F., and Frank A. Sloan, eds. *Organ Transplantation Policy: Issues and Prospects.* Durham, N.C.: Duke University Press, 1989.

Brink, David O. "Moral Conflict and Its Structure." In Mason, *Moral Dilemmas and Moral Theory.*

Callahan, Joan C. "On Harming the Dead," *Ethics,* 97 (January 1987), pp. 341–352.

Caplan, Arthur L., and Daniel H. Coelho, eds. *The Ethics of Organ Transplants.* Amherst, N.Y.: Prometheus Books, 1998.

————, and Beth Virnig. "Is Altruism Enough?—Required Request and the Donation of Cadaveric Organs and Tissues in the United States," *Critical Care Clinics,* 6:4 (October 1990), p. 1017.

Chang, Ruth. *Incommensurability, Incomparability, and Practical Reasoning.* Cambridge, Mass.: Harvard University Press, 1997.

Chang, Ruth. "Introduction." In *Incommensurability, Incomparability, and Practical Reasoning.*

Childress, James, F. "Ethical Criteria for Procuring and Distributing Organs for Transplantation." In *Organ Transplantation Policy: Issues and Prospects.* Edited by James F. Blumstein and Frank A. Sloan. Durham, N.C.: Duke University Press, 1989.

―――. "Organ and Tissue Procurement: Ethical and Legal Issues Regarding Cadavers." In *Encyclopedia of Bioethics.* Edited by Warren T. Reich. New York: Macmillan, 1996.

Cohen, Lloyd R. "Increasing the Supply of Transplant Organs: The Virtues of a Futures Market," *George Washington Law Review,* 1:3 (1989).

Cole, David. "Statutory Definitions of Death and the Management of Terminally Ill Patients Who May Become Organ Donors after Death," *Kennedy Institute of Ethics Journal,* 3:2 (June 1993), pp. 145–155.

Committee on Xenograft Transplantation: Ethical Issues and Public Policy. *Xenotransplantation: Science, Ethics, and Public Policy.* Edited by Division of Health Sciences Policy, Division of Healthcare Services, Institute of Medicine. Washington, D.C.: National Academy Press, 1996.

Condic, Maureen L. "The Basics about Stem Cells," *First Things,* no. 119 (January 2003), pp. 30–34.

Cooper, David K. C., and Robert P. Lanza. *Xeno: The Promise of Transplanting Animal Organs into Humans.* New York: Oxford University Press, 2000.

Council on Ethical and Judicial Affairs, American Medical Association. "Strategies for Cadaveric Organ Procurement: Mandated Choice and Presumed Consent," *Journal of the American Medical Association,* 272:10 (14 September 1994), p. 809.

Daar, A. S. "Ethics of Xenotransplantation: Animal Issues, Consent, and Likely Transformation of Transplant Ethics," *World Journal of Surgery,* 21 (1997), pp. 975–982.

The Decision: Whose Kidney Is It Anyway? FFH 6438. Princeton, N.J.: Films for the Humanities & Sciences, 1996). Film.

DeVita, Michael A., and Ake Grenvik. "History of Organ Donation by Patients with Cardiac Death," *Kennedy Institute of Ethics Journal,* 3:2 (June 1993), pp. 113–129.

―――, and James V. Snyder. "Development of the University of Pittsburgh Medical Center Policy for the Care of Terminally Ill Patients Who May Become Organ Donors after Death Following the Removal of Life Support," *Kennedy Institute of Ethics Journal,* 3:2 (June 1993), pp. 131–143.

Donagan, Alan. "Consistency in Rationalist Moral Systems." In Gowans, *Moral Dilemmas.*

Edinger, John Walter. "The Ethics of Organ Procurement." PhD diss., The University of Texas at Austin, 1987.

Engelhardt, H. Tristram. *Bioethics and Secular Humanism: The Search for a Common Morality.* Laurel, Md.: Trinity Press International, 1991.

————. *The Foundations of Bioethics*. 2nd ed. New York: Oxford University Press, 1996.

————. "Reexamining the Definition of Death and Becoming Clearer about What It Is to be Alive." In Zaner, *Death: Beyond Whole Brain Criteria*, pp. 91–98.

Etzioni, Amitai. "Introduction: A Matter of Balance, Rights and Responsibilities." In *The Essential Communitarian Reader*. Lanham, Md.: Rowman & Littlefield Publishers, Inc., 1998.

Faris, Mickie Hall. *When Your Kidneys Fail*. Los Angeles, Calif.: National Kidney Foundation of Southern California, 1994.

Feinberg, Joel. *Harm to Others: The Moral Limits of the Criminal Law*. New York: Oxford University Press, 1984.

————. "The Mistreatment of Dead Bodies," *The Hastings Center Report*, 15:1 (February 1985), pp. 31–37.

Feldman, Fred. "On the Intrinsic Value of Pleasures," *Ethics*, 107 (April 1997), pp. 448–466.

Fletcher, John. "Human Stem Cell Research: Continued Debate," *American Society for Bioethics and Humanities Exchange*, 2:2 (Spring 1999), p. 7.

Fox, Renee C. "An Ignoble Form of Cannibalism: Reflections on the Pittsburgh Protocol for Procuring Organs from Non-Heart-Beating Cadavers," *Kennedy Institute of Ethics Journal*, 3:2 (June 1993), pp. 231–239.

————, and Judith P. Swazey. "Leaving the Field," *Hastings Center Report*, 22:5 (September–October 1992), pp. 9–15.

————. *Spare Parts: Organ Replacement in American Society*. New York: Oxford University Press, 1992.

Frey, Ray Gillespie "Medicine, Animal Experimentation, and the Moral Problem of Unfortunate Humans." In *Social Philosophy & Policy Foundation*. New York: Cambridge University Press, 1996.

————. "Conflict and Resolution: On Values and Trade-Offs." In Attig et al., *Social Policy and Conflict Resolution*, pp. 1–16.

Geevarghese, S. K., A. E. Bradley, J. K. Wright, et al. "Outcomes Analysis in 100 Liver Transplantation Patients," *American Journal of Surgery*, 175:5 (May 1998), pp. 349–350.

Geron Advisory Ethics Board. "Research with Human Embryonic Stem Cells: Ethical Considerations," *Hastings Center Report*, 29:2 (March–April 1999), pp. 31–36.

Gilligan, Carol. *In a Different Voice: Psychological Theory and Women's Development*. Cambridge, Mass.: Harvard University Press, 1982.

Gowans, Christopher, ed. *Moral Dilemmas*. New York: Oxford University Press, 1987.

Grady, K. L., A. Jalowiec, and, C. White-Williams. "Quality of Life 6 Months after Heart Transplantation Compared with Indicators of Illness Severity Before Transplantation," *American Journal of Critical Care*, 7:2 (March 1998), pp. 106–116.

Greenspan, Patricia S. "Moral Dilemmas and Guilt," *Philosophical Studies*, 43 (1983), pp. 117–125.

————. *Practical Guilt: Moral Dilemmas, Emotions, and Social Norms.* New York: Oxford University Press, 1995.

Griffin, James. "Are There Incommensurable Values?" *Philosophy & Public Affairs,* 7:1 (1977), pp. 39–59.

————. "Incommensurability: What's the Problem?" In Chang. *Incommensurability, Incomparability, and Practical Reason.*

Gross, C. R., M. Malinchoc, W. R. Kim, et al. "Quality of Life Before and After Liver Transplantation for Cholestatic Liver Disease," *Hepatology,* 29:2 (February 1999), pp. 356–364.

Halevy, Amir, and Baruch Brody. "Brain Death: Reconciling Definitions, Criteria, and Tests," *Annals of Internal Medicine,* suppl. 1, 119:6 (15 September 1993), pp. 519–525.

Hetzer, R. et al. "Status of Patients Presently Living 9 to 13 Years after Orthotopic Heart Transplantation," *Annals of Thoracic Surgery,* 64:6 (December 1997), pp. 1661–1668.

Hill, Thomas. "Moral Dilemmas, Gaps, and Residues: A Kantian Perspective." In Mason, *Moral Dilemmas and Moral Theory,* pp. 167–199.

Hooker, Brad. "Ross Style Pluralism versus Rule-Consequentialism," *Mind,* 105 (October 1996), pp. 531–552.

Hughes, Jonathan. "Xenografting: Ethical Issues," *Journal of Medical Ethics,* 24 (1998), pp. 18–24.

Jalowiec, A., K. L. Grady, C. White-Williams, S. Fazekas, M. Laff, V. Davidson-Bell, et al. "Symptom Distress Three Months after Heart Transplantation," *Journal of Heart & Lung Transplantation,* 16:6 (June 1997), p. 611.

Jonas, Hans. *Philosophical Essays: From Ancient Creed to Technological Man.* Chicago, Ill.: The University of Chicago Press, 1974.

Jofre, R., J. M. Lopez-Gomez, F. Moreno, D. Sanz-Guajardo, and F. Valderrabano. "Changes in Quality of Life after Renal Transplantation," *American Journal of Kidney Diseases,* 32:1 (July 1998), pp. 93–100.

Johnson, C. D. "Racial and Gender Differences in Quality of Life following Kidney Transplantation," *Image—The Journal of Nursing Scholarship,* 30:2 (1998), pp. 125–130.

Jonsen, Albert R., Mark Seigler, and William J. Winslade. *Clinical Ethics.* 4th ed. New York: McGraw-Hill, 1998.

Jonsen, Elizabeth, E. Athlin, and O. Suhr. "Familial Amyloidotic Patients' Experience of the Disease and of Liver Transplantation," *Journal of Advanced Nursing,* 27:1 (January 1998), pp. 52–58.

Joralemon, D., and K. M. Fujinaga. "Studying the Quality of Life after Organ Transplantation: Research Problems and Solutions," *Social Science & Medicine,* 44:9 (May 1997), pp. 1259–1269.

Kant, Immanuel. *Grounding for the Metaphysics of Morals.* Translated by James W. Ellington. Indianapolis, Ind.: Hackett Publishing Company, 1981.

Kekes, John. *The Morality of Pluralism*. Princeton, N. J.: Princeton University Press, 1993.

Knowles, Lori P. "Property, Progeny, and Patents," *Hastings Center Report*, 29:2 (March–April, 1999), pp. 38–40.

Lamb, David. "Reversibility and Death: A Reply to David J. Cole," *Journal of Medical Ethics*, 18:1 (1992), pp. 31–33.

Lawrence, Matthew. "Pluralism, Liberalism, and the Role of Overriding Values," *Pacific Philosophical Quarterly*, 77 (1996), pp. 335–350.

Littlefield, C., S. Abbey, D. Fiducia, et al. "Quality of Life Following Transplantation of the Heart, Liver, and Lungs," *General Hospital Psychiatry*, suppl. 6, 18 (November 1996), pp. 37s–47s.

Lynn, Joanne. "Are the Patients Who Become Organ Donors under the Pittsburgh Protocol for 'Non-Heart-Beating Donors' Really Dead?" *Kennedy Institute of Ethics Journal*, 3:2 (June 1993), pp. 167–178.

Mackie, J. L. *Ethics: Inventing Right and Wrong*. New York: Penguin Books, 1977.

Malouin, Rebecca. "Surgeons' Quest for Life: The History and the Future of Xenotransplantation," *Perspectives in Biology and Medicine*, 37:3 (Spring 1994), pp. 416–428.

Marcus, Ruth Barcan. "Moral Dilemmas and Consistency," *Journal of Philosophy*, 77 (1980), pp. 121–136.

Mason, H. E., ed. *Moral Dilemmas and Moral Theory*. New York: Oxford University Press, 1996.

Matas, Arthur J., L. McHugh, W. D. Payne, L. E. Wrenshall, D. L. Dunn, R. W. Gruessner, D. E. Sutherland, and J. S. Najarian, "Long-Term Quality of Life After Kidney and Simultaneous Pancreas-Kidney Transplantation," *Clinical Transplantation,* 12:3 (June 1998), pp. 233–242.

May, William. "Attitudes toward the Newly Dead," *The Hastings Center Studies*, 1:1 (1973), pp. 3–13.

McConnell, Terrance C. "Moral Residue and Dilemmas." In Mason, *Moral Dilemmas and Moral Theory*.

———. "Dilemmas and Incommensurateness," *The Journal of Value Inquiry*, 27 (1993), pp. 247–252.

McGee, Glenn, and Arthur L. Caplan. "What's in the Dish?" *Hastings Center Report*, 29:2 (March–April 1999), pp. 36–38.

Mill, John Stuart. *Utilitarianism*. Indianapolis, Ind.: Hackett Publishing Company, 1979.

Mingardi, G. "Quality of Life and End Stage Renal Disease," *International Journal of Artificial Organs*, 21:11 (November 1998), pp. 741–747.

Monagle, John F., and David C. Thomasma, eds. *Medical Ethics: A Guide for Health Professionals*. Gaithersburg, Md.: Aspen Publishers, 1988.

Mothersill, Mary. "The Moral Dilemmas Debate." In Mason, *Moral Dilemmas and Moral Theory*, pp. 66–85.

Nagel, Thomas. "The Fragmentation of Value." In *Mortal Questions*. New York: Cambridge University Press, 1979.

Neoral Transplant Learning Center. *Your Heart Transplant—Every Step of the Way.* East Hanover, N.J., Norvartis Pharmaceutical Corporation, 1997.

Nietzsche, Friedrich. *Beyond Good and Evil.* New York: Vintage Books, 1966.

O'Carroll, Thomas L. "Over My Dead Body: Recognizing Property Rights in Corpses," *Journal of Health and Hospital Law,* 29:4 (1997), pp. 238–256.

Okarma, Thomas B. "Human Primordial Stem Cells," *Hastings Center Report,* 2:2 (Spring 1999), p. 30.

Paske, Gerald. "Genuine Moral Dilemmas and the Containment of Incoherence," *The Journal of Value Inquiry,* 24:4 (October 1990), pp. 315–323.

Pellegrino, Edmund D. "Families' Self-Interest and the Cadaver's Organs: What Price Consent?" In Caplan and Coelho, *The Ethics of Organ Transplants.*

———, and David C. Thomasma. *The Virtues in Medical Practice.* New York: Oxford University Press, 1993.

Pisani, F., G. Vennarecci, G. Tisone, O. Buonomo, G. Iaria, S. Rossi, A. Famulari, and C. U. Casciani. "Quality of Life and Long-Term Follow-Up after Kidney Transplantation: A 30-Year Clinical Study," *Transplantation Proceedings,* 29:7 (November 1997), pp. 2812–2813.

Pitcher, George. "The Misfortunes of the Dead," *American Philosophical Quarterly,* 21:2 (April 1984), pp. 183–188.

President's Commission for the Study of Ethical Problems in Medicine and Biomedical and Behavioral Research. *Defining Death: A Report on the Medical, Legal and Ethical Issues in the Determination of Death.* Washington D.C.: US GPO, July 1981.

Price, David. *Legal and Ethical Aspects of Organ Transplantation.* New York: Cambridge University Press, 2000.

Radin, Margaret Jane. *Contested Commodities.* Cambridge, Mass.: Harvard University Press, 1996.

Railton, Peter. "Pluralism, Determinacy, and Dilemma," *Ethics,* 102 (July 1992), pp. 720–742.

Rawls, John. *A Theory of Justice.* Cambridge, Mass.: Harvard University Press, 1971.

Regan, Donald. "Value, Comparability, and Choice." In Chang. *Incommensurability, Incomparability, and Practical Reason.*

Reich, Warren T., ed. *Encyclopedia of Bioethics* (New York: Macmillan, 1996).

Rolston, Holmes, III. "The Human Standing in Nature: Fitness in the Moral Overseer." In Sumner et al. *Values and Moral Standing,* pp. 90–101.

Ross, William David. *The Right and the Good.* Oxford: Clarendon Press, 1930.

Rothman, David J. "The International Organ Traffic," *New York Review of Books,* 26 March 1998, pp. 14–17.

Sains, Ariane. "The Stem Cell Frontier," *Europe,* 4:5 (April 2002), p. 28.

Salmon, P., G. Mikhail, S. C. Stanford, S. Zielinsk, and J. R. Pepper, "Psychological Adjustment after Cardiac Transplantation," *Journal of Psychosomatic Research,* 45:5 (November 1998), pp. 449–458.

Sen, Amartya, and Bernard Williams, eds. *Utilitarianism and Beyond*. New York: Cambridge University Press, 1982.

Serafini, Anthony. "Callahan on Harming the Dead," *Journal of Philosophical Research*, 15 (1989–90), pp. 329–339.

Sherwin, Susan. *No Longer Patient: Feminist Ethics & Health Care*. Philadelphia, Pa.: Temple University Press, 1992.

Shewmon, Alan D. "Caution in the Definition and Diagnosis of Infant Brain Death." In Monagle and Thomasma, *Medical Ethics: A Guide for Health Professionals*, pp. 38–57.

Siminoff, Laura A., R. M. Arnold, A. L. Caplan, B. A. Virnig, and D. L. Seltzer. "Public Policy Governing Organ and Tissue Procurement in the United States: Results from the National Organ and Tissue Procurement Study," *Annals of Internal Medicine*, 123:1 (1 July 1995), pp. 10–17.

Siminoff, Laura A., and Alexia Bloch. "American Attitudes and Beliefs about Brain Death." In Youngner et al. *The Definition of Death*, pp. 183–193.

Singer, Peter. *Animal Liberation*. New York: Harper Collins Publishers, 1975.

———. *Rethinking Life and Death: The Collapse of Our Traditional Ethics*. New York: St. Martin's Griffin, 1994.

Sinnott-Armstrong, Walter. *Moral Dilemmas*. Oxford: Basil Blackwell, 1988.

———. "Moral Dilemmas and Rights." In Mason, *Moral Dilemmas and Moral Theory*, pp. 48–65.

Spann, J. C., and C. Van Meter. "Cardiac Transplantation," *Surgical Clinics of North America*, 78:5 (October, 1998), pp. 679–690.

Stocker, Michael. "Abstract and Concrete Value: Plurality, Conflict, and Maximization." In Chang, *Incommensurability, Incomparability, and Practical Reasoning*, 196–214.

———. *Plural and Conflicting Values*. Oxford, England: Clarendon Press, 1990.

Styron, William. *Sophie's Choice*. New York: Bantam Books, 1980.

Sumner, Wayne L., Donald M. Callen, and Thomas Attig, eds. *Values and Moral Standing* (Bowling Green, Ohio: Applied Philosophy Program, Bowling Green State University, 1986).

Tarter, R. E. "Quality of Life Following Liver Transplantation," *Hepato-Gastroenterology*, 45:23 (September–October 1998), pp. 1398–1403.

Taylor, Charles. "The Diversity of Goods." In Sen and Williams, *Utilitarianism and Beyond*, pp. 129–144.

Tomlinson, Tom. "The Irreversibility of Death: Reply to Cole," *Kennedy Institute of Ethics Journal*, 3:2 (June 1993), pp. 157–165.

Tong, Rosemarie. *Feminist Approaches to Bioethics: Theoretical Reflections and Practical Applications*. Boulder, Colo.: Westview Press, 1997.

Transplant Service of the University of Texas Medical Branch at Galveston. *Kidney Transplantation*. Galveston, Tex.: University of Texas, 1998.

Truog, Robert D. "Is It Time to Abandon Brain Death?" *Hastings Center Report*, 27:1 (January–February 1997), pp. 29–37.

———, and James C. Fackler. "Rethinking Brain Death," *Critical Care Medicine*, 20:12 (1992), pp. 1705–1713.

Vanderpool, Harold. "Xenotransplantation: Progress and Promise," *Western Journal of Medicine*, 171 (November/December 1999), pp. 333–335.

———. "Commentary: A Critique of Clark's Frightening Xenotransplantation Scenario," *Journal of Law, Medicine, & Ethics*, 27 (1999), pp. 153–157.

van Fraassen, Bas C. "Values and the Heart's Command," In Gowans, *Moral Dilemmas*, pp. 5–19.

Veatch, Robert M. *Death, Dying, and the Biological Revolution*. 3rd ed. New Haven, Conn.: Yale University Press, 1989.

———. "The Definition of Death: Problems for Public Policy." In Wass et al. *Dying: Facing the Facts*.

———. "The Impending Collapse of Whole Brain Death," *Hastings Center Report*, 23:4 (July–August 1993), pp. 18–24.

———. "Routine Inquiry about Organ Donation—An Alternative to Presumed Consent," *The New England Journal of Medicine*, 325:17 (24 October 1991), pp. 1246–1249.

———. "Whole Brain, Neocortical, and Higher Brain Related Concepts." In Zaner. *Death: Beyond Whole Brain Criteria*, pp. 171–186.

Warren, Mary Anne. *Moral Status: Obligations to Persons and Other Living Things*. New York: Oxford University Press, 2000.

Wass, Hannelore, Robert A. Neimeyer, Felix, M. Berardo, and Francis Taylor, eds. *Dying: Facing the Facts*. 3rd ed. New York: Taylor & Francis Publishing, 1995.

White, Gladys B. "Foresight, Insight, Oversight," *Hastings Center Report*, 29:2 (March–April 1999), pp. 41–42.

Williams, Bernard. *Moral Luck*. New York: Cambridge University Press, 1981.

Wolf, Susan. "Two Levels of Pluralism," *Ethics*, 102 (July 1992), pp. 720–742.

Youngner, Stuart J., Robert M. Arnold, and Renie Schapiro, eds. *The Definition of Death: Contemporary Controversies*. Baltimore, Md.: The Johns Hopkins University Press, 1999.

Younossi, Z. M., and G. Guyatt. "Quality-of-Life Assessments and Chronic Liver Disease," *American Journal of Gastroenterology*, 93:7 (July 1998), pp. 1037–1041.

Zaner, Richard M. "Brains and Persons: A Critique of Veatch's View." In *Death: Beyond Whole Brain Criteria*.

———, ed. *Death: Beyond Whole Brain Criteria*. Dordrect, Holland: Kluwer, 1988.

ABOUT THE AUTHOR

Charles Hinkley teaches philosophy at Texas State University–San Marcos, Texas in the United States. He took the MA in philosophy from Bowling Green State University and the PhD in the medical humanities from the University of Texas Medical Branch at Galveston, Texas. His current research interests include the sources of moral disagreement, preventive medicine, and moral psychology. Along with his research interests, Dr. Hinkley is committed to increasing his anti-war efforts and his support for those suffering from mental illness.

INDEX

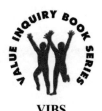

VIBS

The **Value Inquiry Book Series** is co-sponsored by:

Titles Published

1. Noel Balzer, *The Human Being as a Logical Thinker*

2. Archie J. Bahm, *Axiology: The Science of Values*

3. H. P. P. (Hennie) Lötter, *Justice for an Unjust Society*

4. H. G. Callaway, *Context for Meaning and Analysis: A Critical Study in the Philosophy of Language*

5. Benjamin S. Llamzon, *A Humane Case for Moral Intuition*

6. James R. Watson, *Between Auschwitz and Tradition: Postmodern Reflections on the Task of Thinking*. A volume in **Holocaust and Genocide Studies**

7. Robert S. Hartman, *Freedom to Live: The Robert Hartman Story*, Edited by Arthur R. Ellis. A volume in **Hartman Institute Axiology Studies**

8. Archie J. Bahm, *Ethics: The Science of Oughtness*

9. George David Miller, *An Idiosyncratic Ethics; Or, the Lauramachean Ethics*

10. Joseph P. DeMarco, *A Coherence Theory in Ethics*

11. Frank G. Forrest, *Valuemetrics^x: The Science of Personal and Professional Ethics*. A volume in **Hartman Institute Axiology Studies**

12. William Gerber, *The Meaning of Life: Insights of the World's Great Thinkers*

13. Richard T. Hull, Editor, *A Quarter Century of Value Inquiry: Presidential Addresses of the American Society for Value Inquiry*. A volume in **Histories and Addresses of Philosophical Societies**

14. William Gerber, *Nuggets of Wisdom from Great Jewish Thinkers: From Biblical Times to the Present*

130.   Richard Rumana, *Richard Rorty: An Annotated Bibliography of Secondary Literature*. A volume in **Studies in Pragmatism and Values**

131.   Stephen Schneck, Editor, *Max Scheler's Acting Persons: New Perspectives* A volume in **Personalist Studies**

132.   Michael Kazanjian, *Learning Values Lifelong: From Inert Ideas to Wholes*. A volume in **Philosophy of Education**

133.   Rudolph Alexander Kofi Cain, *Alain Leroy Locke: Race, Culture, and the Education of African American Adults*. A volume in **African American Philosophy**

134.   Werner Krieglstein, *Compassion: A New Philosophy of the Other*

135.   Robert N. Fisher, Daniel T. Primozic, Peter A. Day, and Joel A. Thompson, Editors, *Suffering, Death, and Identity*. A volume in **Personalist Studies**

136.   Steven Schroeder, *Touching Philosophy, Sounding Religion, Placing Education*. A volume in **Philosophy of Education**

137.   Guy DeBrock, *Process Pragmatism: Essays on a Quiet Philosophical Revolution*. A volume in **Studies in Pragmatism and Values**

138.   Lennart Nordenfelt and Per-Erik Liss, Editors, *Dimensions of Health and Health Promotion*

139.   Amihud Gilead, *Singularity and Other Possibilities: Panenmentalist Novelties*

140.   Samantha Mei-che Pang, *Nursing Ethics in Modern China: Conflicting Values and Competing Role Requirements*. A volume in **Studies in Applied Ethics**

141.   Christine M. Koggel, Allannah Furlong, and Charles Levin, Editors, *Confidential Relationships: Psychoanalytic, Ethical, and Legal Contexts*. A volume in **Philosophy and Psychology**

142.   Peter A. Redpath, Editor, *A Thomistic Tapestry: Essays in Memory of Étienne Gilson*. A volume in **Gilson Studies**